Nitroglycerin 5

Nitroglycerin 5

Fifth Hamburg Symposium

Edited by Bodo E. Strauer

Walter de Gruyter
Berlin · New York 1987

Responsible for the scientific programme:
Prof. Dr. B. E. Strauer
Division of Cardiology
Department of Internal Medicine
Lahnberge Clinic
Philipps University of Marburg
D-3550 Marburg/Lahn

This book contains 53 illustrations and 9 tables.

CIP-Kurztitelaufnahme der Deutschen Bibliothek

Nitroglycerin ... / ... Hamburg Symposium. – [Engl. Ausg.]. – Berlin ; New York ; de Gruyter
Dt. Ausg. unter demselben Titel
NE: Hamburger Nitroglycerin-Symposium
5. 2nd November 1985. – 1987
ISBN 3-11-010879-8

Library of Congress Cataloging in Publication Data

Hamburg Symposium (5th : 1987)
Nitroglycerin 5.

Includes bibliographies.
1. Nitroglycerin--Therapeutic use--Congresses.
I. Strauer, B. E. (Bodo-Eckehard) II. Title.
III. Title: Nitroglycerin 5. [DNLM: 1. Glyceryl Trinitrate--congresses. 2. Glyceryl Trinitrate--Therapeutic use--congresses. W3 HA177 5th 1985n / QV 156 H199 1985n]
RM666.N725H36 1985 615'.2711 86-24275
ISBN 0-89925-163-3 (U.S.)

 Typesetting and Printing: Buch- und Offsetdruckerei Wagner GmbH, Nördlingen. – Binding: Dieter Mikolai, Berlin. – Cover design: Rudolf Hübler. – Printed in Germany.

Contents

List of contributors

Prof. Dr. W. D. Bussmann
Zentrum der Inneren Medizin
Abteilung für Kardiologie
Klinikum der Johann-Wolfgang-Goethe-Universität Frankfurt
Theodor-Stern-Kai 7
D-6000 Frankfurt/Main 70

Prof. Dr. W. Ehrly
Zentrum der Inneren Medizin
Abteilung Angiologie
Klinikum der Johann-Wolfgang-Goethe-Universität Frankfurt
Theodor-Stern-Kai 7
D-6000 Frankfurt/Main 70

Dr. E. Ernst
Klinik für physikal. Medizin der Ludwig-Maximilians-Universität München
Hämorheologisches Forschungslabor
Ziemssenstr. 1
D-8000 München 2

Priv.-Doz. Dr. N. Fanke
Institut für Anästhesiologie der Ludwig-Maximilians-Universität München
Klinikum Großhadern
Marchioninistr. 15
D-8000 München 70

Prof. Dr. A. G. Franks jr.
60 Gramercy Park North
New York, NY 10010
USA

I. Hutton, M. D.
University Department of Medical Cardiology
Royal Infirmary
Glasgow, G31 2ER

Prof. Dr. H. J. Just
Abt. Innere Medizin III
Klinikum der Albert-Ludwigs-Universität Freiburg
Hugstetter Str. 55
D-7800 Freiburg/Breisgau

Prof. Dr. W. Klaus	Pharmakologisches Institut der Universität Köln Gleueler Str. 24 D-5000 Köln 41
Dr. J. O. Parker	Division of Cardiology Etherington Hall Queens University Kingston, Ontario Canada
Dr. W. Schneider	Pharmakologisches Institut der Universität Wien Währinger Str. 13 a A-1090 Wien
Dr. M. Staritz	I. Med. Klinik und Poliklinik Klinikum der Johann-Gutenberg Universität Mainz Langenbeckstr. 1 D-6000 Mainz
Prof. Dr. M. Stauch	Sektion Kardiologie, Angiologie, Pulmonologie Zentrum für Innere Medizin Universität Ulm Steinhövelstr. 9 D-7900 Ulm
Prof. Dr. M. Tauchert	Medizinische Klinik Stadtkrankenhaus Leverkusen Dhünnberg 60 D-5090 Leverkusen
K. K. Teo, M. D.	Department of Cardiology Saint Laurence's Hospital Dublin 7

Opening remarks

This workshop will deal with some more recent fields of nitroglycerin research. I am particularly happy that a number of foreign guests are present as well. This is why we are having simultaneous translation. I think this is the first time that participants from the United States, Canada and Great Britain have joined us for a nitro symposium. You know that nitroglycerin has a multifactorial effect and acts upon many organs, i.e. not just on the heart, the coronary vascular system, but on the smooth muscles generally. This complexity of nitroglycerin effects means that the programme presented today is also very complex and is broadly based. Because of the numerous nitroglycerin effects it comprises a number of medical disciplines, and this is why speakers from the fields of pharmacology, angiology, then anaesthesiology, dermatology, and finally internal medicine, in particular cardiology and gastro-enterology, have been invited.

Nitroglycerin has been available clinically for more than a hundred years – one is tempted to say on the market – a therapeutic evergreen, and it is surprising that new results are found even now. We shall see what opinions are expressed on this in the papers.

The speakers whom we were able to win are Professor Klaus from Cologne, who is going to make a comparison of nitrates and calcium antagonists in his fundamental paper; then Professor Ehrly from Frankfurt, who is going to present his new and innovative findings in rheology; then the authors Dr. Ernst and Dr. Matrei from Munich continuing with the same subject; then Mr. Franke, a lecturer from Munich, who is an anaesthesiologist and who will focus on microcirculation of the heart, particularly under hypotension and surgical measures; then Professor Franks, a dermatologist from New York, who is going to present the effects of nitrate on the vascular system in conditions of vasospasm and vasculitis in Raynaud's disease; and Dr. Staritz from Mainz with a subject from the field of gastro-enterology under the effect of nitrates in gastro-enterologic indications.

The afternoon will be devoted entirely to the heart. Professor Bussmann from Frankfurt will present his findings on nitroglycerin effects in acute myocardial infarction; Professor Stauch will report on monotherapy and combination therapy with nitrates, the possible combinations. And then there will be the subject of nitrate tolerance which has been hotly debated for years and that Professor Just from Freiburg and Professor Tauchert from Leverkusen will give us their views upon. Afterwards there will be a joint discussion.

Ladies and gentlemen, I should like to open the symposium. I have introduced the speakers to you and now request Professor Klaus to start his fundamental paper on nitrates and calcium antagonists.

B. E. Strauer

Current pharmacology of nitrates and calcium antagonists

W. Klaus

Introduction

The pharmacological basis of the therapeutic effects of organonitrates and calcium antagonists have been described in a number of papers before in such a comprehensive manner [e. g. 3, 10, 17] that, apart from a review of their fundamental mode of action, certain aspects only are to be selected for a more detailed presentation. Although the range of indications for these classes of drugs has been extended to a considerable degree recently, the treatment of coronary failure is still the traditional focus of therapeutic applications to which the following remarks will be confined.

Preliminary remarks on pathophysiology and therapeutic principles of coronary failure

The classical form of exercise-induced angina, based on a fixed arteriosclerotic stenosis of an afferent epicardial coronary vessel, is characterised by the fact that due to impaired functional capacity of the heart muscle at the beginning of the exercise situation, end-diastolic pressure rises drastically and results in regional compression of the subendocardial vascular bed if the reduced poststenotic perfusion pressure is exceeded. The result is subendocardial ischaemia which becomes evident in the ECG as a typical ST-segment depression (fig. 1). As opposed to this, transmural ischaemias (with ST-segment elevation in the ECG) may form through obstruction of a stenotic vessel, for example, by aggregating thrombocytes or superposed vasospastic reactions.

The basic therapeutic approaches (fig. 2) to a functional compensation of these regional disturbances of myocardial oxygen balance are: 1. to lower the overall oxygen demand of the heart by reducing internal and external cardiac performance as is possible by diminishing preload, afterload and heart rate, or 2. to improve poststenotic oxygen supply by eliminating or preventing vasospastic reactions through the interaction with thrombocytes [16] and/or α-adrenergic mechanisms [5]. (Perfusion pressure increases should only be considered in certain special cases).

Nitroglycerin 5

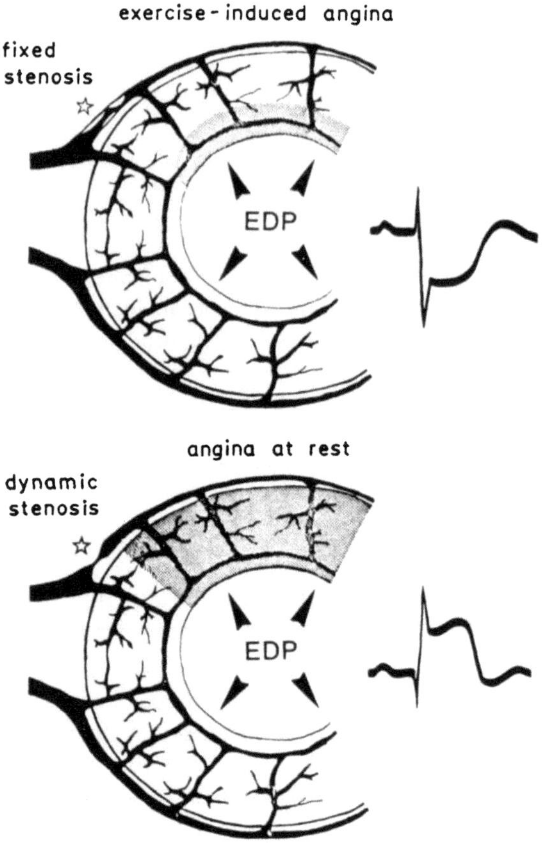

Fig. 1 Schematic representation of the different regional perfusion conditions and ECG-changes in fixed and dynamic coronary stenoses.

Organonitrates and calcium antagonists are capable of influencing individual components to different extents; in principle, both groups of active substances are suitable for this therapeutic aim while their profiles of action have different points of emphasis.

Mode of action of organonitrates

Organonitrates have a relaxant effect on vascular smooth muscles after undergoing intracellular biochemical activation to form a nitrosothiol with SH-group donor involvement (fig. 3). Via stimulation of guanylate cyclase, cGMP is increased;

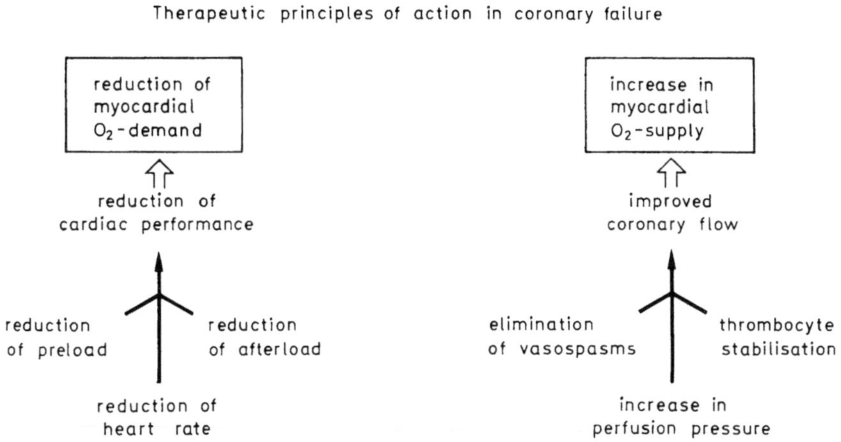

Fig. 2 Therapeutic mode of action in medical treatment of coronary failure.

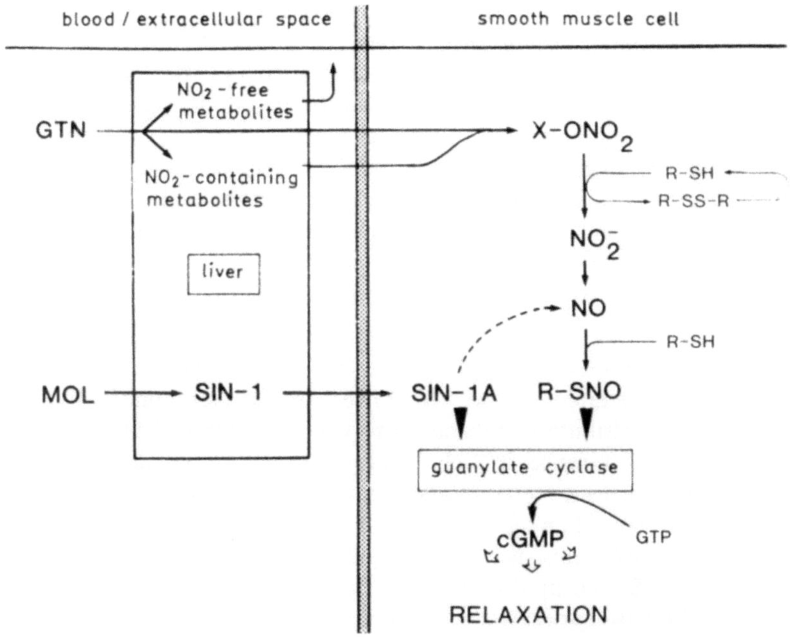

Fig. 3 Comparison of the reaction pathways of nitroglycerin (GTN) with those of molsidomine (MOL) and its metabolites SIN-1 and SIN-1A causing smooth vascular muscle relaxation via activation of guanylate cyclase (based on [1, 6, 7, 9]).

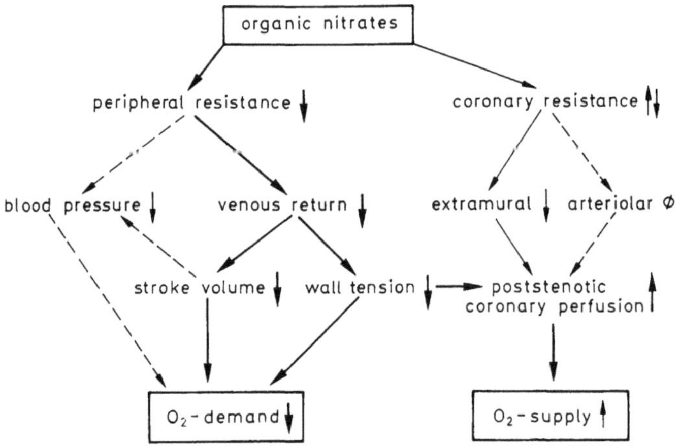

Fig. 4 Schematic representation of the mechanism of action of organic nitrates on myocardial O_2-balance. For details refer to text.

thereby the free calcium concentration is reduced (probably due to stimulation of outward transport) as a result of which vascular tone falls [1, 7]. This effect is known to be much more pronounced in the venous vascular bed than in the arterial one, the consequences being venous pooling, reduced ventricular filling, a decrease in wall tension, in stroke volume and in mean arterial pressure (fig. 4). The reduction in internal and external cardiac performance due to lower preload is associated with a corresponding myocardial oxygen saving. In addition, the drop in end-diastolic pressure has a favourable effect on endocardial perfusion which may, moreover, be improved by dilating effects on the epicardial vessels, certainly if they had an elevated tone before.

The different sensitivities of arterial and venous vessels and the inhomogeneous behaviour of the dose-effect curves (fig. 5) led to the assumption that different mechanisms might contribute to relaxation to varying extents. This was underlined by the quantitative difference in behaviour between arterial and venous vessel preparations during tolerance tests. While in arteries pretreatment with nitroglycerin resulted in a massive weakening of subsequent doses – above all in the low dose range – relaxation of veins was less impaired under comparable conditions. Moreover, by giving SH-group donors (such as cysteine) the tolerance phenomenon (which is said to be based at least in part on depletion of the thiol pool required for intracellular nitrate activation and for this reason is not observed with molsidomine which is independent of thiol) could be compensated in the veins but not in the arteries. While an involvement of prostaglandins in the relaxing effect of low

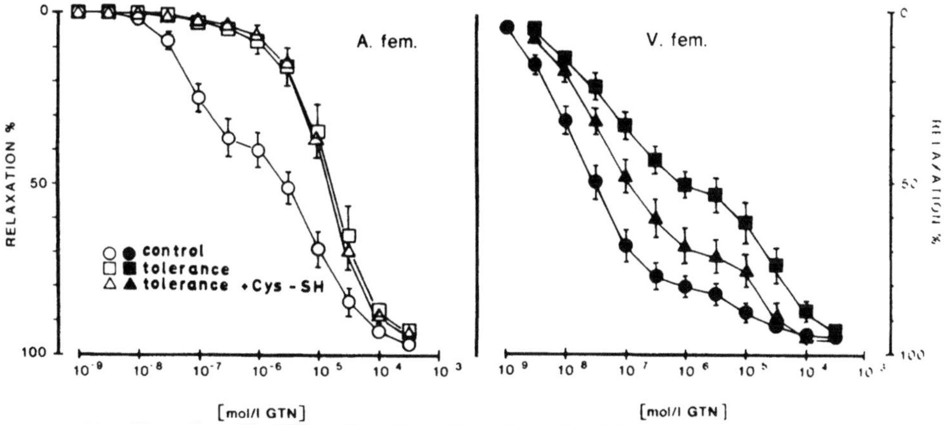

Fig. 5 Concentration dependence of nitroglycerin (GTN)-induced relaxation of vascular preparations before (control) and after action of a high nitroglycerin concentration (GTN, 5×10^{-5} mol/1,60 min) and with addition of cysteine (Cys-SH). For details refer to text [12].

nitroglycerin doses could be substantiated in the arteries (through blockade with indomethacin), this was only related to a relatively minor subcomponent of overall relaxation. Thus the real basis for the different responses of various types of vessel to organonitrates continues to be unclear.

Mechanism of action of calcium antagonists

In contrast to this, the calcium antagonists lead to a decrease in activation of the contractile system in smooth vascular and cardiac muscle (fig. 6) through inhibition of transmembranous calcium inflow. The functional consequences (fig. 7) relevant for therapeutic application relate to the arterial system, e. g. a reduction in afterload, external cardiac performance and thus in myocardial oxygen demand. (Nitrate-like haemodynamic effects, however, can only be induced by much higher doses.) In addition, coronary vascular resistance may be lowered drastically especially in the presence of an excessive vascular tone, the consequence being better poststenotic perfusion and oxygen supply.

The predominant effect on extramural coronary vessels can be identified in videoangiometric measurements, for example in the rabbit heart (fig. 8), demonstrating that

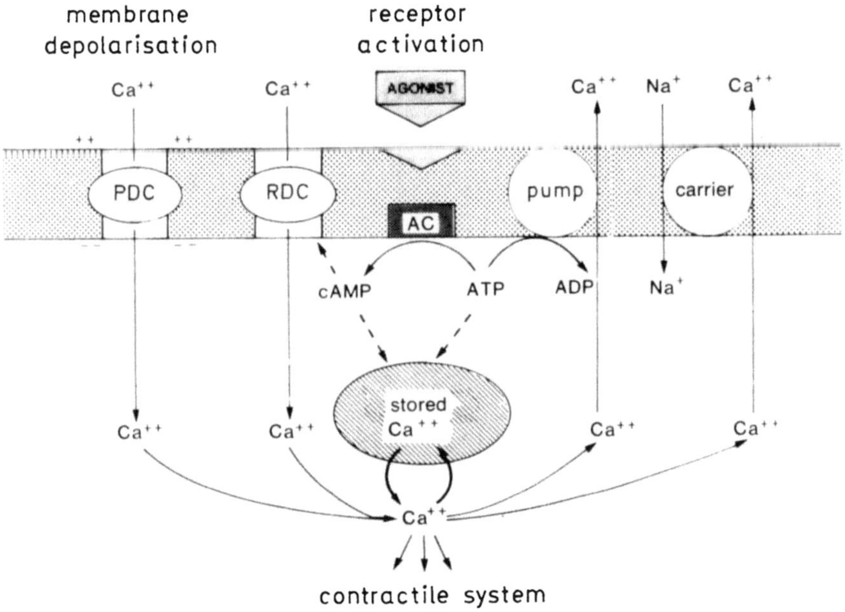

Fig. 6 Schematic diagram of the various mechanism involved in transmembrane calcium passage which govern the concentration of free calcium and thus the activation of the contractile system together with the calcium turnover in intracellular pools. Calcium antagonists tend to block the potential-dependent, to some extent the receptor-dependent channel (PDC and RDC; AC = adenylate cyclase).

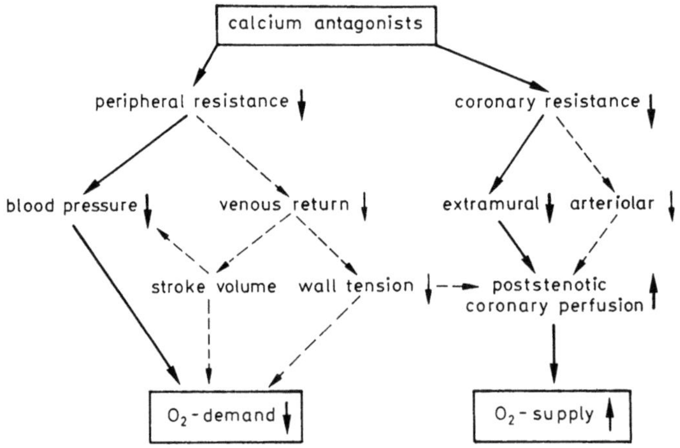

Fig. 7 Schematic representation of the mechanism of action on myocardial O_2-balance of calcium antagonists. For details refer to text.

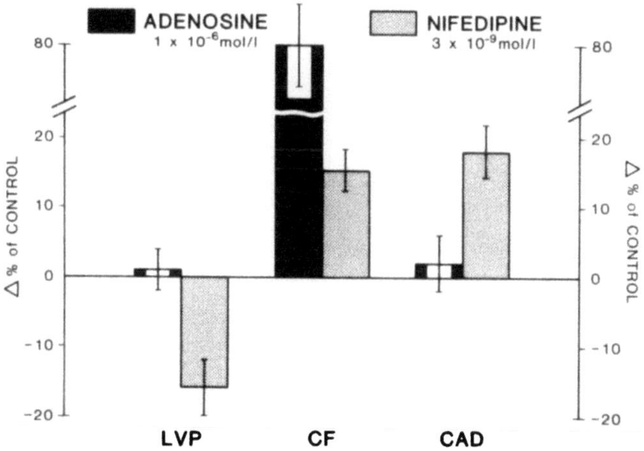

Fig. 8 Comparison of effects of adenosine and nifedipine (at concentrations which do not excessively influence intraventricular pressure (LVP)) on coronary flow (CF) and on the diameter of epicardial coronary arteries (CAD) in isolated rabbit hearts [after 11].

a 20% increase in coronary diameter ensued under nifedipine and not under adenosine – which specifically dilates in the arteriolar region – although nifedipine in the concentration used increased coronary flow much less than adenosine. Thus different segments of the coronary system seem to differ as to their susceptibility to dilating influences, which might also explain the absence of a steal phenomenon after application of calcium antagonists (as opposed to adenosine-mediated coronary dilation).

The specific vasodilative quality of calcium antagonists is furthermore documented by experiments in coronary ligated rabbit hearts. Even in persisting ligation the subsequent administration of calcium antagonists resulted in a distinct decrease of the ischaemic region (measured by epicardial NADH fluorescence as a parameter of tissue oxygenation) which can only be explained by a marked action on the collateral vessels (fig. 9).

Influencing eicosanoid-dependent functions in thrombocytes and vascular wall

In addition to the direct vascular effects achieved by organonitrates and calcium antagonists, their possible influence on platelet function and their interaction with

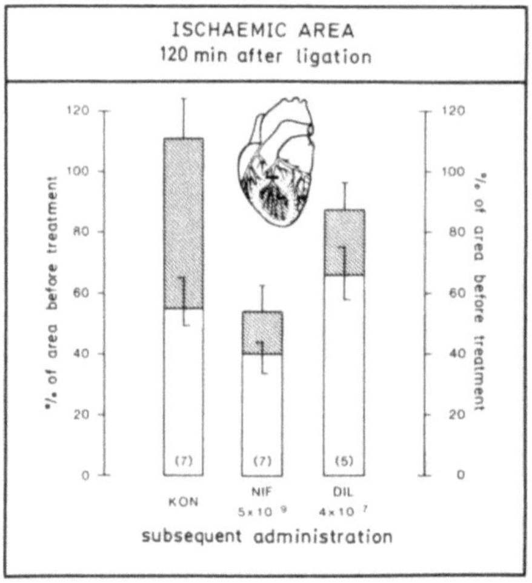

Fig. 9 Extent of ischaemic area (determined by epicardial NADH fluorescence) following coronary ligation of the isolated rabbit heart; without treatment (CON) and with subsequent administration of nifedipine (NIF) or diltiazem (DIL). The proportion of severe ischaemia is shaded [after 13].

the vascular bed has recently met with some special interest [4, 15]. When arachidonic acid metabolism is stimulated, different endproducts with opposing qualities develop in platelets and the vascular wall (fig. 10): in the thrombocytes thromboxane is formed and this further activates thrombocyte aggregation via a positive feedback mechanism (among other things by inducing the release of vasoactive spasmogens such as serotonin and 12-HPETE) and which causes vasoconstriction when acting on vascular smooth muscle. On the other hand, prostacyclin, which has antiaggregational and vasodilative properties, originates in the vascular wall (mainly from the endothelium). If the intima is damaged, the normally existing balance between these two functional antagonists is shifted in favour of thromboxane; hypothetically therefore, locally elevated thrombocyte aggregation is induced with narrowing of the vascular diameter and secretion of vasospastic components which may cause an increase in vascular tone. In the presence of an existing eccentric atheromatous stenosis, for instance, this might lead to critical narrowing. The involvement of such a mechanism in the development of vasospastic pectanginal conditions is accentuated by the favourable therapeutic effects of thrombocyte aggregation inhibitors (like acetylsalicylic acid) in patients with unstable angina pectoris [8].

In order to investigate any intrinsic activity of the organonitrates and calcium antagonists in respect of the mediators involved in those pathophysiological events

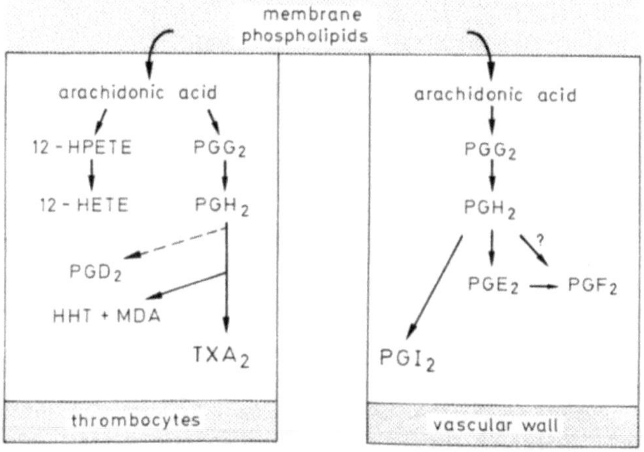

Fig. 10 Schematic representation of arachidonic acid metabolism in thrombocytes and the vascular wall.

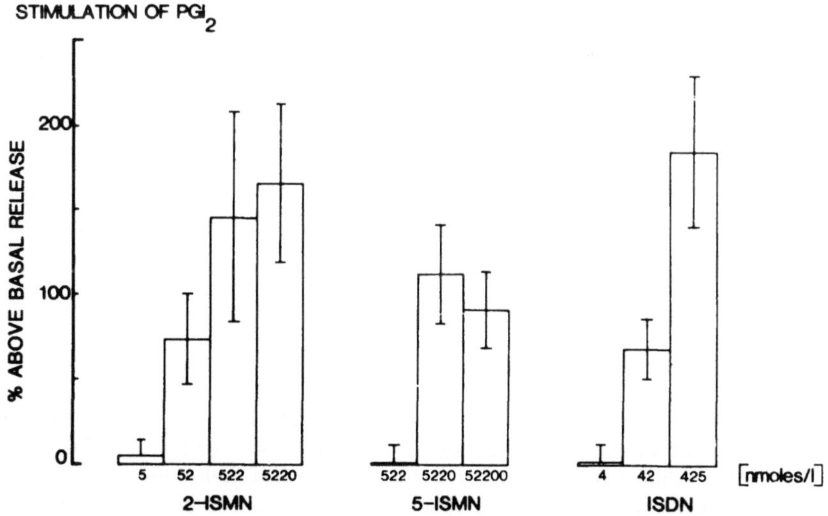

Fig. 11 Concentration-dependent incrase in prostacyclin (PGI_2) formation in isolated coronary arteries induced by isosorbide dinitrate (ISDN) and isosorbide mononitrate (2-ISMN, 5-ISMN), [after 14].

PARAMETER	GTN	SIN-1	NIF
thrombocyte aggregation	○	↓	(↓)
PGI_2 formation	↑	○	○
TXA_2 formation	○	↓	(↓)
12-HPETE formation	○	↓	?

Fig. 12 Influence on thrombocyte aggregation, vascular prostacyclin formation, thrombocytic thromboxane and 12-HPETE formation by nitroglycerin (NTG), the active metabolites of molsidomine (SIN-1) and nifedipine (NIF), (after data from [2, 14]).

provoking vasospasms, both kinds of drugs were applied to thrombocytes and vascular muscle preparations. As indicated in figs. 11 and 12, nitroglycerin and other organonitrates stimulated vascular prostacyclin formation concentration-dependently (while thrombocytic functions were not influenced directly), whereas the active metabolite of molsidomine (which did not have any impact on vascular prostacyclin formation) stabilised the thrombocytes. Nifedipine, on the other hand, had only platelet inhibition effects (requiring greater than therapeutic concentrations in vitro, although the relevant in vivo studies document efficacy antagonists). It can be assumed, therefore, that all of these agents used for treating coronary insufficiency have – besides their vasodilatative effect – additional favourable consequences for the interaction between thrombocytes and the vascular wall. The clinical importance of this effect, however, cannot yet be assessed in comparison with the haemodynamic relief and the lowering of coronary tone.

References

[1] Boehme, E., G. Grossmann, C. Spies: Effects of molsidomine and other NO-containing vasodilators on cyclic GMP-formation. Eur. Heart. J. **4,** Suppl. C. (1983) 19–24.

[2] Darius, H., Ahland B., Rücker W. et al.: The effects of molsidomine and its metabolite SIN-1 on vessel tone, platelet aggregation and eicosanoid formation in vitro. J. Cardiovasc. Pharmacol. **6** (1984) 115–121.

[3] Fleckenstein A.: Calcium Antagonism in Heart and Smooth Muscle. John Wiley & Sons, New York 1983.

[4] Hammersen, F., E. Hammersen: Zur funktionellen Morphologie des Endothels unter besonderer Berücksichtigung der Koronargefäße. Z. Kardiol. **74,** Suppl. 7 (1985) 73–77.

[5] Heusch, G., A. Deussen: The effects of cardiac sympathetic nerve stimulation on perfusion of stenotic coronary arteries in the dog. Circ. Res. **46** (1980) 426–429.

[6] Ignarro, L. J., H. Lippton, J. C. Edwards et al.: Mechanism of vascular smooth muscle relaxation by organic nitrates, nitrites, nitroprusside and nitric oxide: evidence of the involvement of N-nitrosothiols as active intermediates. J. Pharmacol. Exp. Ther. **218** (1981) 759–749.

[7] Kukovetz, W. R., S. Holzmann: Mechanism of nitrate-induced vasodilation and tolerance. Z. Kardiol. **72**, Suppl. 3 (1983) 14–19.

[8] Lewis, H. D., J. M. Davis, D. G. Archibald et al.: Protective effects of aspirin against acute myocardial infarction and death in men with unstable angina. New Engl. J. Med. **309** (1983) 396–403.

[9] Needleman, P.: Organic nitrate metabolism. Ann. Rev. Pharmacol. **16** (1976) 81–93.

[10] Opie, L. H. (ed.): Calcium Antagonists and Cardiovascular Disease. Raven Press, New York 1984.

[11] Rösen, R., J. W. Sielemann, W. Klaus: Action profile of adenosine and nifedipine on arterial vessels in isolated heart preparations. Pflüger's Arch. Eur. J. Physiol. **402,** Suppl. (1984) R 27.

[12] Rösen, R., E. König, W. Klaus: Comparative analysis of glyceryltrinitrate (GTN) induced relaxation in different types of vessels. Naunyn Schmiedeberg's Arch. Pharmacol. **329,** Suppl. (1985) R 59.

[13] Rösen, R. B. Kleuren, A. Heider et al.: Change of NADH-surface-fluorescence by nifedipine and diltiazem in locally ischemic rabbit hearts. J. Mol. Cell. Cardiol. **17,** Suppl. 3 (1985) 89.

[14] Schrör, K., B. Ahland, H. Darius et al.: Stimulation of vascular PGI_2 by organic nitrates and its significance for the antianginal effect. Scand. J. Clin. Lab. Invest. **44,** Suppl. 173 (1984) 33–38.

[15] Schrör, K., Prostaglandine and Endothelzellen. Z. Kardiol. **74,** Suppl. 7 (1985) 93–97.

[16] Shepherd, J. T., P. M. Vanhoutte: Spasm of the coronary arteries: Causes and consequences (the scientist's viewpoint). Mayo Clin. Proc. **60** (1985) 33–46.

[17] Sorki, E. M., R. N. Brogden, J. A. Romankiewicz: Intravenous glyceryl trinitrate (nitroglycerin). A review of its pharmacological properties and therapeutic efficacy. Drugs **27** (1984) 45–80.

[18] Stiefel, A., V. A. W. Kreye: On the hemodynamic differences between sodium nitropruside, nitroglycerin, and isosorbide nitrates. Naunyn-Schmiedeberg's Arch. Pharmacol. **325** (1984) 270–274.

Effects and modes of action of nitrates upon rheologic properties of the blood and the supply to ischaemic tissue

A. M. Ehrly

Introduction

In addition to classical therapy of angina pectoris with organic nitrates, an attempt has been made in the past few years to treat certain forms of chronic occlusive arterial disease by systemic or local application of nitrates. With regard to the mode of action, the vasodilative property of nitroglycerin and other nitrates has been known for many decades. Moreover, cardiac work is reduced by decreasing afterload. Hossmann et al. [1] reported in 1982 that in addition blood viscosity can be reduced through nitrates. In 1983 Ehrly and Landgraf [2] found in detailed studies that after the administration of 20 mg isosorbide dinitrate to patients with intermittent claudication, not just whole blood viscosity but also plasma viscosity is reduced as a function of time. Erythrocyte filterability and erythrocyte aggregation, however, only tend towards a reduction which is not significant statistically. With regard to the mechanism of action involved in reducing whole blood viscosity, both Hossmann and Cäsar and our group suspected internal, i.e. endogenous, haemodilution. The assumption is that after giving nitrates an improvement in perfusion and a decrease in peripheral resistance is not just due to vasodilation, but also to a reduction in internal friction of the blood, i.e. blood viscosity.

The above results have given rise to more questions. For example, it seemed interesting to find what mechanism induces internal haemodilution with lowering of blood and plasma viscosity after administration of nitrates. The question of whether through vasodilation and a simultaneous reduction in blood viscosity the supply to ischaemic tissue areas is improved or not is more important, because it is more relevant clinically. We know from peripheral occlusive diseases that as a rule vasodilation alone will lead to increased perfusion in healthy tissue areas but to reduced perfusion in ischaemic tissue areas. It is known, moreover, from animal experiments by Schroeder et al. [3] that increased perfusion due to vasodilation is inhomogeneous, i.e. that short bridge capillaries have a perfusion surplus while the longer so-called nutritional capillaries are perfused less. It was shown that, on balance, the supply to tissue deteriorates despite elevated overall perfusion. Since in ischaemic diseases there is inhomogenous capillary perfusion by definition (maldis-

Nitroglycerin 5

tribution [4, 5]), it is conceivable that additional drug induced vasodilation will further increase this inhomogeneity of capillary perfusion while deteriorating further supply to tissue.

In order to clarify the first question relating to the mechanism of action of endogenous, internal, or autohaemodilution, our group carried out a number of experimental studies which I do not want to talk about in detail. In principle, it can be stated that according to these studies the rheological properties of the blood change at the same time as vascular diameters in the microcirulation; this we have called rheoregulation [6, 7]. It means that peripheral resistance and thus capillary perfusion is also a function of synchronous changes in blood viscosity when vessel diameters are changed. We demonstrated that the administration of sympathomimetic agents, such as etilefrin, results in both vasoconstriction and an increase in haematocrit readings with a simultaneous rise in blood and plasma viscosity [8]. The same applies to the infusion of noradrenaline [9]. Emotional stress also leads to an increase in blood and plasma viscosity via haemoconcentration [10, 11]. Vasodilators such as isosorbide dinitrate [2], on the other hand, result in vasodilation, and as was explained above, additionally to a drop in blood and plasma viscosity. The previously mentioned studies suggest that through measures of vasoconstriction, as well as of vasodilation at the periphery, the isogravimetric point is shifted, as a result of which the equilibrium changes between external filtration of fluid from the intravascular space into the interstitial space and reabsorption from the interstitial space into the intravascular space. Detailed information on this mechanism of rheoregulation has been given elsewhere [6, 7].

However, the critical question, of whether an improved supply to tissue, in particular to ischaemic areas, can be achieved by vasodilation and a simultaneous reduction in blood and plasma viscosity can on no account be clarified through extra vivum studies (and that is what rheologic studies are), but only through a quantitative determination of tissue supply direct in ischaemic tissues. One measurement technique available for this is to determine tissue oxygen pressure by polarography [12]. In the case of organic nitrates direct quantification on the ischaemic heart muscle would of course be desirable; this has not been possible to date, however, for technical reasons. For our studies we therefore selected patients with intermittent claudications at stage IIb in whom anatomical and pathophysiological conditions, it is true, do not correspond directly to those prevailing in coronary heart disease, but they have some pathogenetic and therapeutic aspects in common. The following part of this paper is to report on studies aimed at investigating changes in rheologic blood properties and in muscle tissue oxygen pressure among patients with intermittent claudication before and after oral administration of isosorbide dinitrate.

Patient population and methods

In 9 patients with chronic occlusive arterial disease at stage IIb tissue oxygen pressure was measured before and after the oral administration of 20 mg isosorbide dinitrate. The investigations were conducted in a supine position and at rest; through an indwelling cannula blood samples were drawn from the cubital vein for rheologic investigation. Measurement of tissue oxygen pressure was made by coated micro-platinum needle electrodes with a tip diameter of 1–3 μm [12]. Following intracutaneous Scandicain-induced anaesthesia, Braun's syringe was put through the skin at the middle of the lower leg, but without reaching the fascia. The outside plastic cover was cut off from Braun's syringe and served as a guide rail for the electrode proper. By means of a micromanipulator this electrode was slowly pushed forward 10 to 12 mm into the anterior tibial muscle. When it was withdrawn with a hydraulic micromanipulator, a continuous measurement was made across the entire length with current variations in the nanoampere range being recorded as a curve. Subsequently, the curve was analysed by a computer, the different pO_2-values (400–500 per mm of tissue) were grouped into classes, and a frequency analysis (a so-called histogram) was made. After 2 blank values, measured with a 15-minute interval, 20 mg ISDN were given orally. After 15, 30, 60, and 120 minutes further measurements of the tissue oxygen pressure were carried out.

At the same times blood pressure and pulse were registered automatically. From the withdrawn blood, whole blood viscosity and plasma viscosity were determined at 37° with a capillary viscosimeter after Ostwald. Furthermore, the haematocrit reading (microhaematocrit centrifuge) was determined, also total RBC in the whole blood and erythrocyte filtration (method after Ehrly and Roßbach), total RBC passing through the filter within five minutes being a yardstick for erythrocyte filtrability. Moreover, erythrocyte aggregation was checked by application of transmission optics after Ehrly and Schmitt, as well as the rate of erythrocyte sedimentation after Westergren. All results were analysed statistically with the Wilcoxon test.

Results

Initial values for the patients with intermittent claudication at stage IIb were about 7 torr for tissue oxygen pressure (tab. 1). No later than 15 minutes after the drug was taken the tissue oxygen pressure rose to 10 torr, which was not, however, statistically significant. 30 and 60 minutes after the tables were administered the mean was still about 10 torr; after 60 minutes there was a statistically significant difference compared to blank data. 120 minutes after the tablets were taken, the pO_2-level was 9 torr, thus approaching initial values again. When analysing the behaviour of pO_2

after giving ISDN you find that the rise in tissue oxygen pressure started at different times, earlier or later, after the tablet was taken depending on the subject. In one patient there was a fall in oxygen pressure within a minimum 30 minutes after administration of the tablet. However, systolic blood pressure also clearly dropped from 180 mmHg to around 40 mmHg in this patient. Apart from this patient, all others had some lowering of systolic blood pressure although not to a statistically significant extent.

The measurements of haemorheologic parameters yielded the known reduction in whole blood viscosity and plasma viscosity with a lower haemotocrit reading. Erythrocyte aggregation levels were mildly reduced in a statitically insignificant manner. Nor were there any statistically significant changes in erythrocyte filtration (see tab. 1).

Table 1 Behaviour of various parameters of measurement before and after acute oral administration of 20 mg Isosorbide dinitrate

	base line values		after oral administration of Isosorbide dinitrate			
	01	02	15 min	30 min	60 min	120 min
muscle tissue pO_2	9,06	8,89	10,74	9,90	10,18*	9,01
($\bar{x} \pm SD$)	6,12	7,15	5,56	5,22	6,62	2,41
RR	155/88	162/88	152/92	148/91	140/91	138/90
($\bar{x} \pm SD$)	18/7	20/7	20/12	19/12	14/12	11/9
blood viscosity $H_{20} = 1$	4,80	4,70	4,64*	4,58	4,58*	4,61*
($\bar{x} \pm SD$)	0,51	0,52	0,53	0,54	0,49	0,48
plasma viscosity $H_{20} = 1$	1,81	1,79	1,77	1,76*	1,77	1,77
($\bar{x} \pm SD$)	0,09	0,07	0,07	0,07	0,06	1,07
hematocrit (%)	42,95	42,40	41,67	41,44	41,22	41,17*
($\bar{x}$*SD)	3,95	3,92	3,62	3,59*	3,97*	3,89

(mean value ± standard deviation; * = statistically significant $2\alpha \leq 0,05$)

Discussion

The investigations show that after administration of ISDN to patients with chronic occlusive arterial disease there is a mean rise in tissue oxygen pressure, which is not statistically significant until 60 minutes after taking the tablets. Behaviour of tissue oxygen pressure following medication is not homogeneous as regards the time of pO increase. When individual levels are analysed, the fact is striking that tissue oxygen pressure only rose slightly or in fact fell below initial levels whenever blood pressure levels clearly dropped within the framework of therapy; such a relationship between systemic blood pressure and tissue oxygen pressure is known. The investigations into the impact of ISDN on tissue oxygen pressure demonstrate that in those patients who do not have a clear drop in blood pressure an improvement in oxygen supply to ischaemic lower leg muscles can certainly be achieved. In principle this is in agreement with studies of an increase in flow through the extremities after ISDN because, as stated above, the absolute level of flow/time volume across an extremity (global blood flow) does not throw any light upon whether nutritional flow is improved or whether a microcirculatory steal phenomenon is the consequence (maldistribution [4, 5]). This is why measurement of tissue oxygen pressure is important as a quantitative parameter of tissue supply.

Our investigations show that in the final analysis there is an improved tissue supply in at least a majority of patients. The present levels of tissue oxygen pressure obtained in the muscles of the lower leg and under resting conditions in patients with intermittent claudication naturally cannot be applied safely to the situation in the tissue of the beating ischeamic heart muscle. In the context of clinical experience the data obtained nevertheless allow you to draw the guarded conclusion that even in impaired coronary blood flow the administration of nitrates will lead to an improved supply to the tissue provided the local pressure gradients are not too pronounced due to an important decrease in systemic blood pressure.

The data gathered on changes in rheologic properties of the blood are in precise agreement with findings published before. Whether and to what extent this reduction in blood and plasma viscosity plays a part in the region of lower leg muscles or, for that matter, in an ischaemic heart muscle cannot be estimated. In theory improved perfusion should result specifically in the low flow areas of microcirculation by means of which nutrition of tissues can be optimized. By measuring tissue oxygen pressure you obtain a final quantity for nutritive tissue supply from which you cannot infer certain mechanisms directly. Examples from the literature show that an improvement in flow properties of the blood need not inevitably lead to an improved supply to tissues.

Summary

Under ISDN there is an improvement in supply to the tissue of lower leg muscles in patients with intermittent claudication if the systemic blood pressure drop is limited. Compared to exogenous haemodilution with plasma substitutes, flow properties of the blood are improved modestly. This might, however, be a contributory factor towards increasing flow values and improving tissue supply. In terms of pathophysiology it is interesting to note that, despite vasodilation in most patients, supply to the tissue does not deteriorate, i.e. that an existing maldistribution in ischaemic diseases at least in the lower leg muscles is not aggravated but reduced.

References

[1] Hossmann, V., H. Wegener, B. Wegener, et al.: Hämorheologische und hämodynamische Wirkungen von Isosorbiddinitrat bei essentieller Hypertonie und arterieller Verschlußkrankheit. In: Nitrate III – kardiovasculäre Wirkungen (H. J. Engel, A. Schrey, P. R. Lichtlen, eds.), p. 287. Springer Verlag, Berlin – Heidelberg – New York 1982.

[2] Ehrly, A. M., H. Landgraf.: Einfluß von Isosorbiddinitrat auf die Fließeigenschaften des Blutes von Patienten mit chronisch arterieller Verschlußkrankheit. In: Therapie mit hämorheologisch wirksamen Substanzen (A. M. Ehrly, ed.), p. 145. Verlag Zuckschwerdt, München 1986.

[3] Schroeder, W.: Die Messung des Sauerstoffdruckes in der Skelettmuskulatur – eine quantitative Methode zur Kontrolle der Sauerstoffversorgung und der Funktion der terminalen Muskelstrombahn. Herz/Kreislauf **10** (1978) 146–153.

[4] Ehrly, A. M., W. Schroeder: Zur Pathophysiologie der chronischen arteriellen Verschlußerkrankung. I. Mikrozirkulatorische Blutverteilungsstörung in der Skelettmuskulatur. Herz/Kreislauf **11** (1979) 275.

[5] Ehrly, A. M.: New pathophysiological concept of ischemic diseasses: Microcirculatory Blood Maldistribution (MBM). Anatomica **20** (1980) 456.

[6] Ehrly, A. M.: Rheoregulation: Influence of vasoconstriction and vasodilation on the flow properties of blood. Abstractband der 4. Europ. Conf. on Clinical Hemorh. Siena 1985.

[7] Ehrly, A. M.: Rheoregulation: Zeitsynchrone Veränderungen der Fließeigenschaften des Blutes in Abhängigkeit vom Sympatikotonus. Vortrag 4. Jahrestagung der Dt. Ges. f. Klin. Hömorheologie, Minden 1985 (im Druck).

[8] Ehrly, A. M.: Einfluß von Etilefrin auf die Fließeigenschaften des Blutes von Patienten mit Claudicatio intermittens (in Vorbereitung).

[9] Takeda, N., T. Kubo, T. Matsunaga, et al.: Effects of Noradrenaline Infusion on the whole blood viscosity and viscosity's regulatory factors. Gibi-inkota Rinsho **7b** (Suppl. 4) (1983) 2308.

[10] Ehrly, A. M., H. Landgraf, J. Heßler, et al.: Influence of a videofilm – induced emotional stress on the flow propertees of blood. Clinical Hemorheology **3** (1983) 254 (Abstract).

[11] Ehrly, A. M., H. Landgraf, J. Heßler, et al.: Influence of a videofilm – induced emotional stress on the flow properties of blood. Vortrag 6. Int. Congr. of Biorheology, Vancouver/ Kanada 1986 (in Vorbereitung).

[12] Ehrly, A. M., H.-J. Köhler, W. Schroeder, et al.: Sauerstoffdruckwerte im ischämischen Muskelgewebe von Patienten mit chronischen peripheren arteriellen Verschlußkrankheiten. Klin. Wochenschr. **53** (1975) 687.

Recent findings on the effect of nitroglycerin on haemorheology

E. Ernst, A. Matrai

Introduction

The literature provides indications that nitrates modify haemorheological parameters. In principle such a mechanism could contribute to the anti-ischaemic effect on the heart [6]. It therefore seemed appropriate to carry out a placebo-controlled double blind study on this complex of questions. The object of this investigation was to clarify whether transdermal and/or sublingual medication with glycerol nitrate induces haemorheological effects in healthy test persons.

Material and methods

The study comprised eleven persons (8 women, 3 men, average age 27 ± 3 years) shown clinically, in terms of their histories and by laboratory tests to be in good health. At 8.00 hrs the first blood sample was taken from each test person under standardized conditions. Then a skin plaster (nitroglycerin or placebo) was applied to the inside of the forearm in a randomized manner. After this the test person was to go about his usual daily routine. After 3 hours a second blood sample was taken, and after 24 hours a third. At least a week later the test person was called in again and the second plaster was applied by analogous procedure. The verum was a 20 cm^2 Nitroderm TTS® plaster with 50 mg glycerol nitrate; the placebo was identical in appearance. After a further two-day washout phase another blood sample was taken. Following this the test persons had to bite open a capsule containing 0.8 mg glycerol nitrate (Nitrolingual®). Two hours later a further blood specimen was taken.

The following parameters were quantified: blood viscosity (BV) at 0.7; 2.4 and 95^{s-1} (37°C) in the LS 30 viscometer (Contraves) [11]; plasma viscosity (PV) and serum viscosity (SV) in the Harkness capillary viscometer at 37°C [16]; colloid osmotic pressure in plasma (PCOP) and in serum (SCOP) (Gonotec Osmomat) [12]; packed cell volume (PCV) (impedance method) [18]; haemoglobin (Hb) (photometrically); erythrocyte and leucocyte counts (TOA cell counter); erythrocyte filterability (EF)

Nitroglycerin 5

[5]; erythrocyte aggregation (EA) (Myrenne) [10]; total protein in serum (biuret method).

The results were evaluated statistically with the Wilcoxon ranking test [27]. The null hypothesis would be rejected if $p < 0.05$.

Results

In the crossover study only the three-hour values could be evaluated statistically as the great majority of the test persons ($n = 10$) had taken the plaster off prematurely because of servere haedaches (on average after 13 ± 5 hours). Three hours after application of the verum plaster the following significant changes were recorded: PV, SV, PCOP, SCOP, PCV and Hb (tab. 1). Analogous changes to the means are recognizable in the data from the 24-hour measurements, which were not tested for significance (tab. 2). Under placebo none of the parameters altered significantly. In

Table 1 Changes (in percent) after three-hour transdermal application

Parameter	Initial values		Changes in % after 3 hours	
	Placebo	Nitro	Placebo	Nitro
BV F = 94.5 l/s	4.53 ± 0.36	4.53 ± 0.46	98 ± 4%	96 ± 5%
F = 2.4 l/s	13.3 ± 2.2	13.1 ± 2.5	93 ± 10%	92 ± 8%
F = 0.7 l/s	22.4 ± 4.6	21.6 ± 4.9	91 ± 10%	90 ± 12%
PV (mPa.s)	1.14 ± 0.03	1.16 ± 0.04	100 ± 2%	99 ± 3%*
SV (mPa.s)	1.06 ± 0.01	1.08 ± 0.03	101 ± 2%	99 ± 2%*
EF	61 ± 4	64 ± 7	97 ± 9%	104 ± 8%
EA	16.3 ± 4.5	17.4 ± 4.5	105 ± 20%	102 ± 17%
PCOP (mmHg)	25.3 ± 1.5	26.3 ± 1.7	102 ± 4%	96 ± 5%*
SCOP (mmHg)	25.1 ± 1.6	26.2 ± 1.8	103 ± 6%	95 ± 7%*
Leucocytes ($10^3/\mu l$)	6.0 ± 1.0	6.4 ± 2.0	115 ± 23%	105 ± 12%
PCV	0.43 ± 0.03	0.44 ± 0.04	100 ± 2%	94 ± 6%*
HB (g/l)	149 ± 15	151 ± 17	100 ± 6%	95 ± 5%**
Erythrocytes ($10^6/l$)	4.72 ± 0.48	4.80 ± 0.52	99 ± 4%	96 ± 7%
Total protein (g/l)	71 ± 3	72 ± 2	99 ± 4%	98 ± 5%

* statistically significant $p < 0.05$

** statistically significant $p < 0.01$

Table 2 Changes (in percent) after 24 hours transdermal application

Parameter	Initial values		Changes in % after 24 hours	
	Placebo	Nitro	Placebo	Nitro
BV F = 94.5 l/s	4.53 ± 0.36	4.53 ± 0.46	97 ± 5%	96 ± 7%
F = 2.4 l/s	13.3 ± 2.2	13.1 ± 2.5	93 ± 11%	95 ± 17%
F = 0.7 l/s	22.4 ± 4.6	21.6 ± 4.9	92 ± 13%	94 ± 22%
PV (mPa.s)	1.14 ± 0.03	1.16 ± 0.04	100 ± 3%	99 ± 2%
SV (mPa.s)	1.06 ± 0.01	1.08 ± 0.03	101 ± 2%	99 ± 3%
Ef	61 ± 4	64 ± 7	95 ± 2%	98 ± 7%
EA	16.3 ± 4.5	17.4 ± 4.5	92 ± 16%	106 ± 14%
PCOP (mmHg)	25.3 ± 1.5	26.3 ± 1.7	99 ± 7%	96 ± 8%
SCOD (mmHg)	25.1 ± 1.6	26.2 ± 1.8	99 ± 9%	96 ± 8%
Leucocytes (10^3/μl)	6.0 ± 1.0	6.4 ± 2.0	108 ± 21%	108 ± 16%
PCV	0.43 ± 0.03	0.44 ± 0.04	101 ± 6%	94 ± 6%
Hb (g/l)	149 ± 15	151 ± 17	101 ± 5%	96 ± 8%
Erythrocytes (10^6/l)	4.72 ± 0.48	4.80 ± 0.52	101 ± 6%	97 ± 8%
Total protein (g/l)	71 ± 3	72 ± 2	99 ± 5%	98 ± 6%

The figures could not be evaluated statistically.

the open part of the test there were significant changes in the parameters: SV, SCOP, and PCV following sublingual administration of glycerol nitrate (tab. 3).

Discussion

Hossman et al. [17] recorded a fall in blood viscosity in patients suffering from occlusive arterial disease after 20 mg ISDN. Ehrly et al. [9] found under analogous conditions that blood viscosity fell up to 2 hours post medicationem. This was largely due to a fall in packed cell volume, as plasma viscosity was only reduced significantly as compared to the initial values after 30 minutes.

The data from our study confirm these earlier findings and show that there is a significant fall in PV, SV, PCOP, SCOP, PCV and Hb after a three-hour transdermal application of glycerol nitrate. The 24-hour measurements which were not evaluated statistically are evidence that these are protracted effects. The single sublingual application induced singificant changes in the parameters, SV, SCOP and PCV after

Table 3 Changes (in percent) after sublingual administration of nitroglycerin

Parameter	Sublingual Nitroglycerin Before	After
BV F = 94.5 l/s	4.2 ± 0.4	97 ± 2%
F = 2.4 l/s	11.2 ± 2.3	94 ± 5%
F = 0.7 l/s	17.8 ± 4.3	92 ± 7%
PV (mPa.s)	1.15 ± 0.03	99 ± 1%
SV (mPa.s)	1.06 ± 0.02	99 ± 2%
EF	60 ± 8	101 ± 10%
EA	16.4 ± 4.1	100 ± 11%
PCOP (mmHg)	23.8 ± 1.7	97 ± 4%
SCOP (mmHg)	23.8 ± 1.4	97 ± 3%**
Leucocytes ($10^3/\mu l$)	6.3 ± 1.3	100 ± 13%
PCV	0.40 ± 0.03	94 ± 5%*
Hb (g/l)	143 ± 12	97 ± 4%
Erythrocytes ($10^6/l$)	4.56 ± 0.40	97 ± 4%
Total protein (g/l)	68 ± 3	99 ± 2%

* statistically significant $p < 0.05$
** statistically significant $p < 0.01$

2 hours. The "autohaemodilution" underlying these changes may be a secondary result of nitrate-induced arterial and venous vasodilatation [14]. Distension proximal and distal to the exchange vessels may reduce capillary filtration pressure which, according to Starling's Law, would lead to a predominance of re-absorption and thus to a redistribution of fluid with an expansion of intravascular volume [26]. It has also been postulated [22] that in the capillary system fluid relatively low in cells and protein stagnates in non-perfused areas without taking part in the systemic circulation. In principle a nitrate-induced re-inclusion of this volume of fluid in the circulation might provide another explanation for the "autohaemodilution". It is a matter for discussion whether the increase in blood fluidity, discrete in healthy persons possibly more apparent in patients, is one of the factors involved in the anti-ischaemic effects of the nitrates. Haemodilution leads to a reduction of the viscous part of resistance [7] and an increase in the venous return [15]. Whatever the underlying mechanism, this can bring about an increase in perfusion and an improvement in oxygen supply [6]. The anti-ischaemic nitrate effects are largely caused by haemodynamic changes for which a reduction in the oxygen requirement of the left ventricle is a necessity. The most important cause of this is systemic venous dilatation

[21]. It seems, however, that an improvement in the myocardial oxygen supply and a redistribution of blood flow in the ischaemic area also have a part to play [19]. It was possible to objectify increased perfusion of collaterals [2] and a redistribution of the blood supply to benefit ischaemic and subendocardial regions [28]. There may be at least a partial connection between improved collateral blood supply and microcirculatory redistribution on the one hand and the "autohaemodilution" described here on the other. This would mean that venous dilatation is the most important anti-ischaemic effect leading to a reduction in oxygen requirements. It seems, however, that haemorheological effects are provoked at the same time, and that these might lead to an increase in the cardiac oxygen supply. In other words: there are several ways in which the nitrate effect leads to a favourable influence on the balance between oxygen supply and demand. This hypothesis could be of relevance to clinical therapy in a manner that has so far received little attention, although it clearly requires further experimental testing.

Summary

Eleven healthy volunteers were treated transdermally with glycerol nitrate or a placebo in a double blind crossover study, then sublingually in an open study. Blood samples were taken before and 3 and 24 hours after the beginning of medication, or 2 hours after medication respectively. Measurements were made of blood, plasma and serum viscosity, colloid osmotic pressure in plasma and serum, erythrocyte flexibility, erythrocyte aggregation, blood count and total protein. Transdermal and sublingual application of glycerol nitrate is followed by haemodilution and an improvement in blood fluidity. In principle this could work synergistically with the known action of nitroglycerin to increase the anti-ischaemic effect.

References

[1] Anderson, C. H., P. Hueber, C. Sterlin et al.: Effects of nitroglycerine on prostacyclin production in rat aorta. Circulation **62** (1980) 326.

[2] Cohen, M. V., J. M. Downey, E. H. Sonnenblick et al.: The effects of nitroglycerin on coronary collaterals and myocardial contractility. J. Clin. Invest. **52** (1973) 1836.

[3] De Caterin, R., D. Giannessi, F. Crea et al.: Antiplatelet effects of isosorbide dinitrate in man. Z. Kardiol. **73**/Suppl. 3 (1983) 46.

[4] De Caterina, R., D. Giannessi, F. Crea et al.: Inhibition of platelet function by injectable isosorbide dinitrate. Am. J. Cardiol. **53** (1984) 1683.

[5] Dodds, J., J. A. Dormandy et al.: Haemorheological response to plasma exchange in Raynaud's Syndrome. Brit. Med. J. **2** (1979) 1186.

[6] Dormandy, J., E. Ernst, A. Matrai et al.: Haemorheological changes following acute myocardial infarction. Am. Heart. J. **104** (1982) 1364.
[7] Dormandy, J., C. Yates, A. Berent et al.: Increase in leg blood-flow by normovolaemic haemodilution in intermittent claudication. Lancet **2** (1979) 166.
[8] Dowd, P. M., J. B. Kovacs, C. J. H. Bland et al.: Effects of prostaglandisn I_2 and E on red cell deformability in patients with Raynaud phenomenon and sustemic sclerosis. Brit. med. J. **283** (1981) 350.
[9] Ehrly, A. M., H. Landgraf: Einfluß von Isosorbiddinitrat auf die Fließeigenschaften des Blutes von Patienten mit chronischer arterieller Verschlußkrankheit. In: Therapie mit hämorheologisch wirksamen Substanzen (A. M. Ehrly, ed.). W. Zuckschwerdt, München 1984.
[10] Ernst, E.: Erythrozyten-Aggregation statt BKS? Labor Praxis **18** (1984).
[11] Ernst, E.: Practical rheology. Med. Focus **3** (1983) 30.
[12] Ernst, E., A. Matrai: Messung des kolloidosmotischen Druckes mit dem Osmomat 050 (Gonotec). Labor Praxis (Nov. 1984) 20–22.
[13] Ernst, E., A. Matrai et al.: Methodological and intraindividual variations in some hemorheological tests. Clin. Hemorheol. **5** (1985) 511–514.
[14] Ferrer, M. J., S. E. Bradley, H. O. Wheeler et al.: Some effects of nitroglycerin upon splanchnic, pulmonary and systemic circulations. Circulation **33** (1966) 357.
[15] Guyton, A. C., T. W. Richardson: The effect of hematocrit on venous return. Circ. Res. **9** (1961) 157.
[16] Harkness, J.: A new instrument for the measurement of plasma viscosity. Lancet **2** (1963) 280.
[17] Hossmann, V., H. Wegener et al.: Hömorheologische und hämodynamische Wirkungen von Isosorbiddinitrat bei essentieller Hypertonie und arterieller Verschlußkrankheit. In: Nitrate III – kardiovaskuläre Wirkungen (H. J. Engel, A. Schrey, P. R. Lichtlen, eds.), pp. 287. Springer, Berlin – Heidelberg 1982.
[18] Kernen, J. A., H. Wurzer, R. Odada: New method of measuring hematocrit: a clinical evaluation. J. Lab. Clin. Med. **57** (1981) 635.
[19] McGregor, M.: Pathogenesis of angina pectoris and role of nitrates in relief of myocardial ischemia. Am. J. Med. **74** (suppl. 6B) (1983) 21.
[20] Levin, R. J., E. A. Jaffe, B. B. Weksler et al.: Nitroglycerin stimulates synthesis of prostacyclin by cultured human endothelial cells. J. Clin Invest. **57** (1981) 762.
[21] Luomanmaki, K.: Efficacy of different forms of nitrates in angina pectoris. Acta Med. Scand. (suppl.) **694** (1984) 153.
[22] Matrai, A., E. Ernst, J. Dormandy: Die Rolle der Hämorheologie in der Medizin unter besonderer Berücksichtigung der Therapie mit β-Blockern. In: Rheologie und β-Blocker (E. Heilmann, H. Kiesewetter, E. Ernst, eds.). Zuckschwerdt, München 1984.
[23] Metha, P., J. Metha: Comparative effects of nitroprusside and nitroglycerin on platelet aggregation in patients with heart failure. J. Cardiovasc. Pharmacol. **2** (1980) 25.
[24] Schafer. A. J., R. W. Alexander, R. J. Handin: Inhibition of platelet function by organic nitrate vasodilators. Blood **5** (1980) 649.
[25] Schror, K., L. Grodzinska, H. Darius et al.: Stimulation of prostaglandin (PGI_2) and inhibition of human platelet thromboxan A_2 after low dose nitroglycerin. Circulation **64** (1981) 283.

[26] Starling, E. H.: On the absorption of fluids from the connective tissue spaces. J. Physiol. **19** (1896) 312.
[27] Weber, E.: Grundriß der biologischen Statistik. G. Fischer, Stuttgart 1980.
[28] Winbury, M. M.: Redistribution of left ventricular blood flow produced by nitrolgycerin. Circulation Res. **1** (1971) 140.

Nitroglycerin therapy in operative medicine considering micro- and macrohaemodynamic aspects

N. Franke

In operative medicine, therapy with nitroglycerin (NTG) plays an important part. The main reason for this fact is that today patients are operated on with cardiac risk factors (e.g. coronary heart disease) and at a high age.

Ranges of indications for therapy with NTG during the perioperative period are:
1. reduction in blood pressure;
2. improvement of myocardial function by diminishing afterload of the right and left heart;
3. therapy of pulmonary oedema by diminishing preload;
4. therapy of acute moycardial ischaemia.

A reduction in blood pressure, improvement of myocardial function and diminishing of preload and afterload can also be achieved through the administration of other vasodilative drugs, e.g. sodium nitroprusside [5, 9]. Although myocardial oxygen demand is reduced as a result, it is not associated with an improvement of regional myocardial oxygen balance in each and every case [2].

The unique effect of NTG on myocardial oxygen balance suggests that NTG does not just act on the greater circulation but also on microcirculation [1]. This is of critical importance since any improvement of haemodynamics in the greater circulation is rather pointless unless it is associated with an improved perfusion of nutritional capillaries and thus an undisturbed exchange of oxygen and substrate in the tissue.

Recent findings on the effects of sodium nitroprusside and NTG on the capillary system and tissue oxygenation in the organs [5, 8] gave rise to detailed investigations into the effects both drugs have on microcirculation. It was striking to find out that nitroprusside-induced hypotension is always accompanied by deterioration of tissue oxygenation [5, 8]. Since tissue hypoxia – measured with an oxygen multi-wire surface electrode on skeletal muscle, the liver, and subcutaneous tissue – occurs despite unobstructed overall flow through the organs [8], it must be due to a change in microcirculatory perfusion. This caused a more detailed study of changes, in the region of the capillary system with nitroprusside-induced hypotension, to be made.

If an aluminium chamber is implanted in a dorsal skin fold of a golden hamster for observation of microcirculation [3], tissue hypoxia can be demonstrated under

Nitroglycerin 5

enflurane anaesthesia and hypotension from nitroprusside (figs. 1 and 2). When blood pressure is lowered with NTG, the bell shape of pO_2-histograms is preserved; the hypoxic and anoxic pO_2-levels ranging from 0–5 mmHg in particular just show a slight increase. Analyses of microhaemodynamics and capillary perfusion only became possible when intravital microscopy was combined with quantitative video techniques. It appeared that in sodium nitroprusside-induced blood pressure reduction, both for 70 mmHg and for 40 mmHg, there is a highly significant drop in density of erythrocyte-perfused capillaries (fig. 3) in the hamster skin muscle. Total organ perfusion remains unchanged because 54% of the blood flowing into microcirculation through arterioles, at a pressure of 40 mmHg, perfuses arteriovenous shunts and therefore flows past the nutritional capillaries. When measuring microvascular

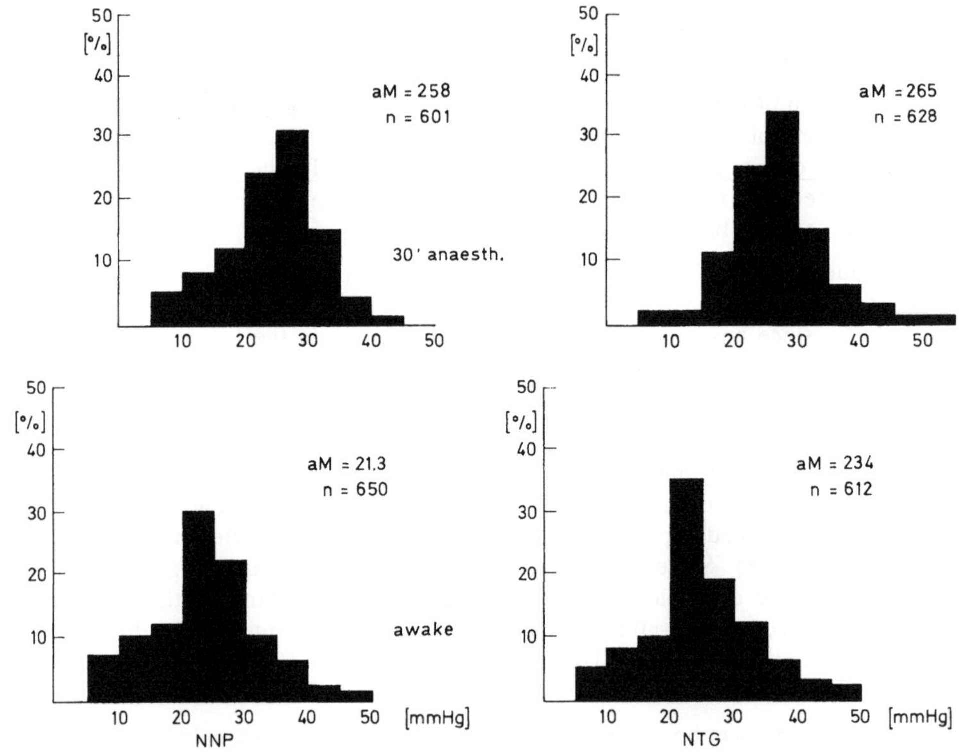

Fig. 1 Frequency distribution of local tissues; pO_2-levels before, during and after enflurane anaesthesia (the NNP and NTG groups are shown separately). aM = arithmetic mean; n = number of individual determinations.

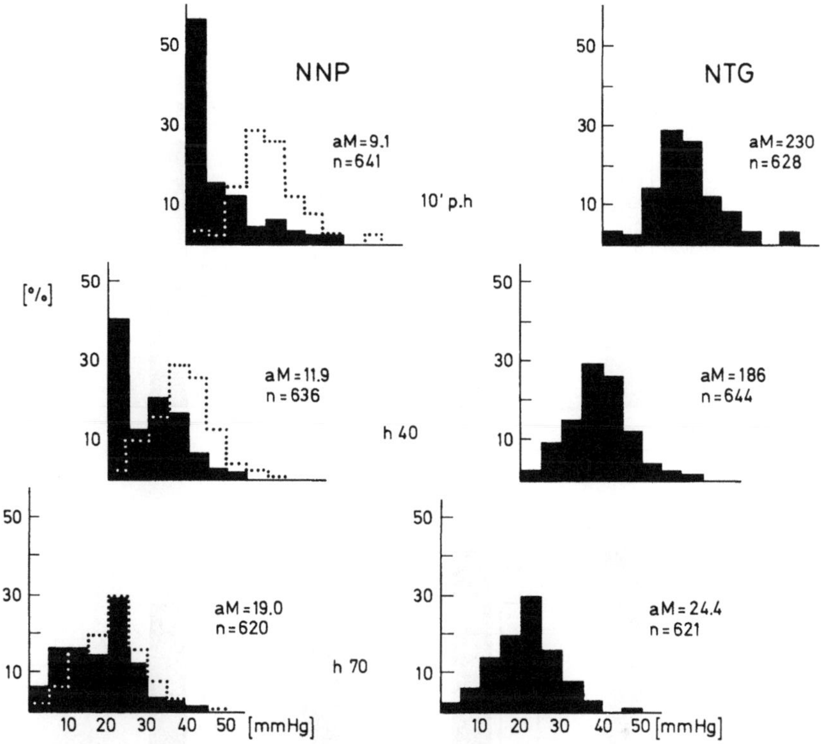

Fig. 2 Frequency distribution of local tissues; pO_2-levels for NNP- und NTG-induced hypotension (dotted = histograms of NTG-induced hypotension; h 70 = moderate hypotension of 70 mmHg, h 40 = severe hypotension of 40 mmHg, 10′ p.h. = 10 minutes after the end of NNP of NTG infusion).

diameters it appears that sodium nitroprusside only dilates the precapillaries while leaving the venules unaffected in the microcirculation (fig. 4). This has important consequences for those pressures in microcirculatory vessels which influence flow. Only arteriolar pressure will fall by 25% to 40 mmHg when sodium nitroprusside is used to reduce pressure. In the collecting venules, however, the pressure rather tends to rise (fig. 5). The reduction of the pressure difference affecting flow between precapillaries and venules results in a redistribution of blood in microcirculation, with a preference for flow through vessels with the lowest possible perfusion resistance (AV shunts).

In NTG-induced moderate and severe hypotension, on the other hand, tissue oxygenation – measured with an oxygen multiwire electrode on the skin chamber

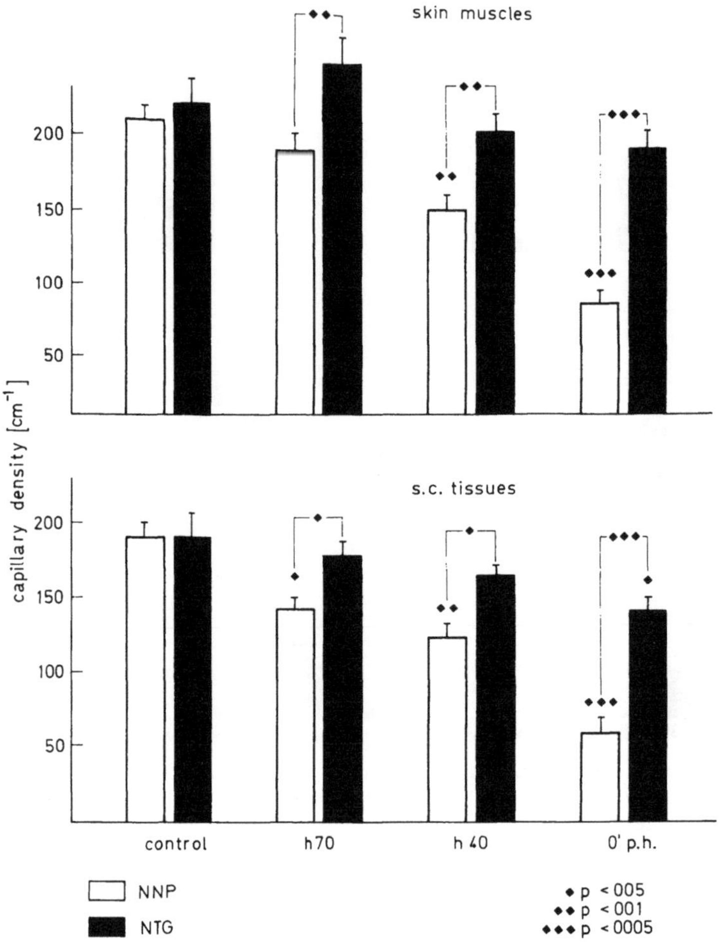

Fig. 3 Change in density of erythrocyte-perfused capillaries during and after NNP- and NTG-induced hypotension (for explanation, see fig. 29.

preparation of the hamster-remains unchanged (figs. 1 and 2). An analysis of microcirculation by intravital microscopy reveals that the density of erythrocyte-perfused capillaries is the same under hypotension (fig. 3). NTG dilates all microcirculatory vessel segments (fig. 4). In moderate and severe hypotension, pressures in the arterioles and venules fall (fig. 5). This is why the pressure gradient affecting flow between arterioles and collecting venules remains unchanged. Therefore, there is no need to divert blood away from nutritional capillaries towards AV shunts.

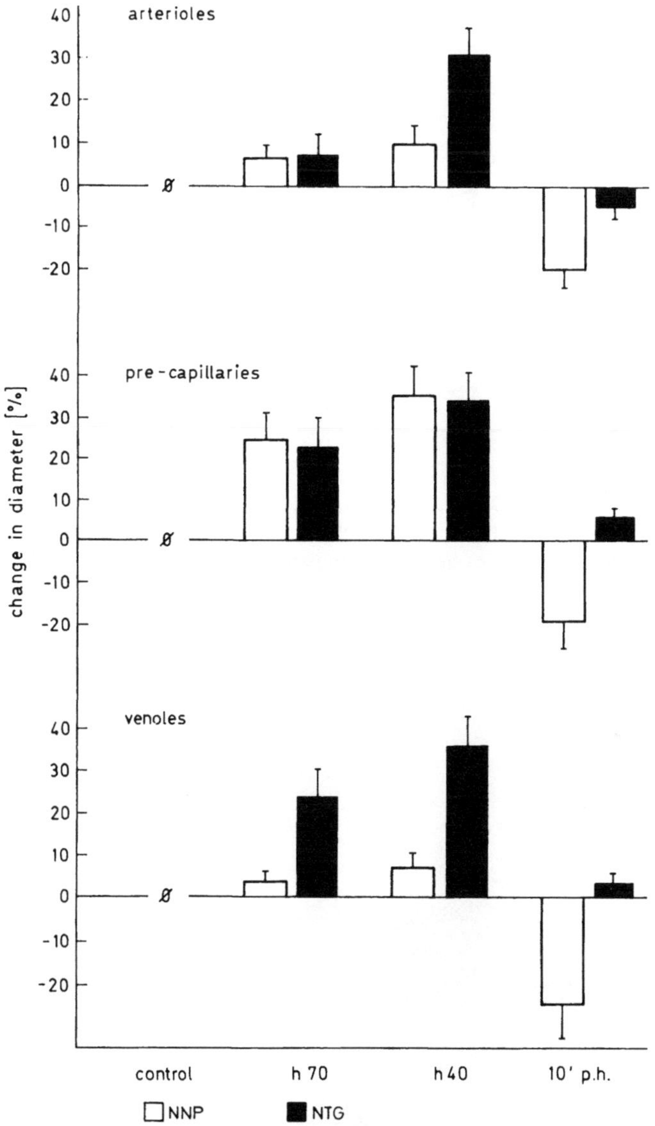

Fig. 4 Manometer changes as a percentage of initial levels in arterioles, precapillaries and venules during and after NNP- and NTG-induced hypotension (for explanation, see fig. 2).

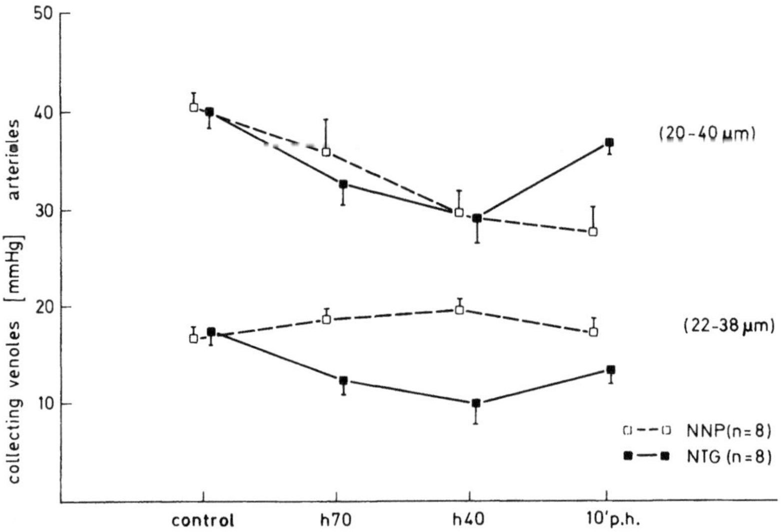

Fig. 5 Pressures in arterioles and venules before, during and after NNP and NTG hypotension (for explanation, see fig. 2).

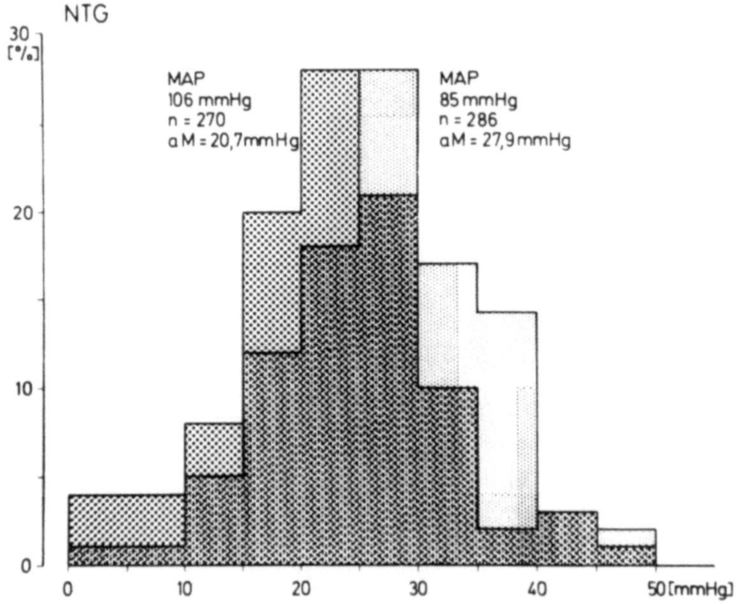

Fig. 6 The influence of moderate NNP-induced blood pressure reduction on the local pO_2-levels (for explanation, see fig. 1).

Some indications of how important these findings are for man are derived from the fact that pronounced tissue hypoxia can be detected on human limb muscle during sodium nitroprusside-induced blood pressure reduction to 85 mmHg (fig. 6). By contrast, improved tissue oxygenation is found when inducing the same hypotension with NTG (fig. 7). This may be explained by better blood flow distribution in the microcirculation.

The influence of NTG on the perfusion of myocardial microcirculation is of particular importance [10]. Following intravenous injection of NTG (30 mg/kg) in the cat and rat, pressure will fall in the aorta, arterioles and venules. The distances between perfused capillaries in the myocardium, however, are significantly reduced following NTG application; so capillary density rises. This suggests a better oxygen supply to the myocardium after the administration of NTG. In addition to the well-known systemic effects of NTG, such as a decrease in preload and afterload 82] with a resultant diminution of myocardial oxygen consumption, this drug apparently leads to specific improvement of myocardial microcirculation.

Similar studies of changes in the microcirculation of heart muscle after giving sodium nitroprusside administration do not yet exist, but it is well known that sodium

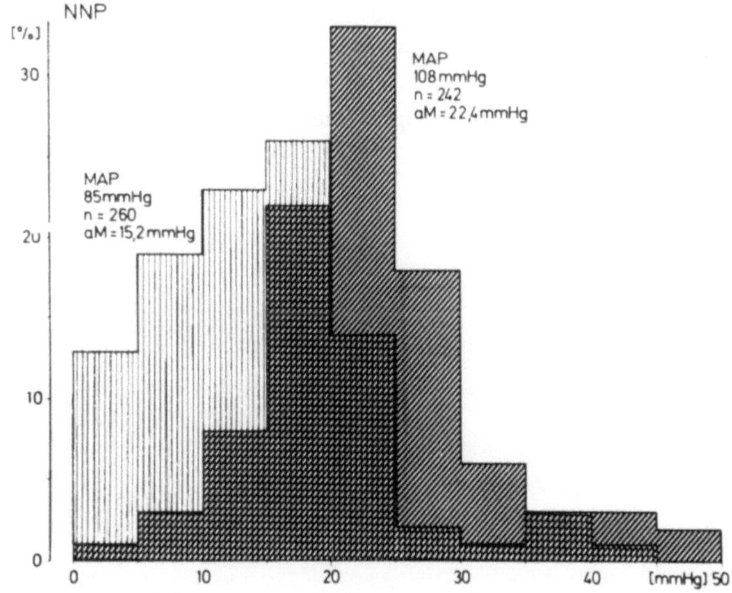

Fig. 7 In moderate hypotension with NTG the local pO_2-levels are improved (for explanation, see fig. 1).

nitroprusside further diminishes regional blood flow through ischaemic areas of the mycardium [3]. Its effect on systemic circulation – diminishing preload and afterload [9] – is similar to that of NTG and leads to lower myocardial oxygen consumption, too. But in the coronary patient, greater ST-segment increases in the ECG following sodium nitroprusside infusion can be detected, whereas in the NTG-induced hypotension there is improved regional perfusion of ischaemic myocardial areas with a decrease in ST-segment depression.

Changes in blood flow through the heart and in myocardial oxygen consumption also indicate that there is a redistribution of flow through the myocardial capillary system. If blood flow in the coronary sinus is measured by means of thermodilution and myocardial oxygen consumption calculated, after both NTG and sodium nitroprusside infusion, the myocardial oxygen consumption decreases in the coronary patient (fig. 8). In these patients, flow in the coronary sinus, that is blood flow through the myocardium, increases after sodium nitroprusside, while the arterio-venous difference in oxygen content is reduced. Together with a drop in myocardial oxygen consumption, blood flow through the myocardium is diminished moderately after NTG while the arterio-venous difference in oxygen content rises moderately. This suggests that in coronary patients, following sodium nitroprusside, the blood flows through the healthy myocardial regions at a high rate and is directed past poststenotic vessels and ischaemic myocardial areas (coronary steal syndrome). Contrary to this situation, it can be assumed that, following the administration of NTG, coronary blood is predominantly supplied to poststenotically undersupplied areas of the myocardium.

The results of these microcirculatory changes, after giving NTG, suggests that it is sensible to use this substance at the perioperative stage in patients at cardiac risk.

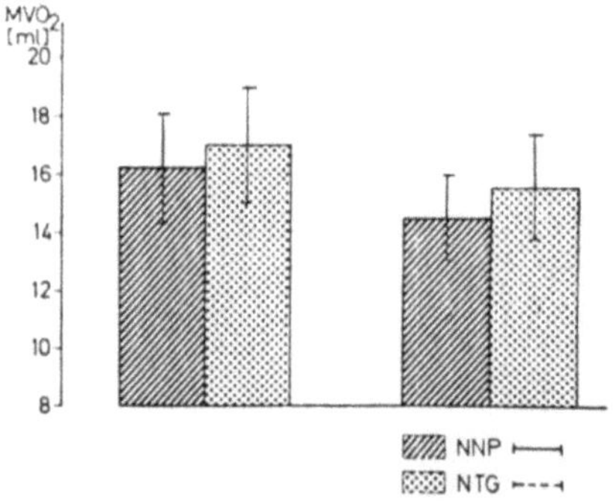

Fig. 8 NNP and NTG cause myocardial oxygen consumptionto fall in a similar way in moderate hypotension.

Whenever possible, NTG should be applied to improve cardiac function by diminishing afterload of the left or right ventricle. In acute hypertension during an operation, moreover, a blood pressure reduction should be induced with NTG if at all possible. If the extent of hypotension is insufficient, other hypotensives, such as urapidil, can be used.

The application of NTG can prevent both nutritional undersupply to tissues and adverse consequences developing from this.

References

[1] Braunwald, E.: Heart disease, p. 550. W. B. Saunders Co., Philadelphia – London – Toronto 1980.

[2] Chatterjee, K., H. J. C. Swan: Vasodilator therapy in acute myocardial infarction. Mod. Con. Cardiov. Dis. **43** (1974) 119.

[3] Endrich, B., A. Ashaihi, K. Goetz: A new chamber technique for microvascular studies in unanesthetized animals. Res. Exp. Med. **177** (1980) 125.

[4] Franke, N., K. van Ackern, K. Peter et al.: Die Wirkung von Natriumnitropussid auf die Hämodynamik von herzgesunden und linksinsuffizienten Patienten. Prakt. Anästh. **13** (1978) 513.

[5] Hauss, J., K. Schönleben, U. Spiegel et al.: Die kontrollierte Hypotension mit Natriumnitropussid. Herz/Kreislauf **10** (1978) 379.

[6] Khambatta, H. J., J. G. Stone, E. Khan: Hypertension during anesthesia on discontinuation of sodium nitropusside-induced hypotension. Anesthesiologie **51** (1979) 127.

[7] Kessler, M., M. Grunewald: Possibilities of measuring oxygen pressure fields in tissue by multivire platinum electrodes. Prog. Respir. Res. **3** (1969) 147.

[8] Meßmer, K., W. J. Stelter, S. Stippig: Sodiumnitroprusside induced hypotension: Flow distribution and metabilism. Eur. Surg. Res. **10**, Supp. 1 (1978) 51.

[9] Palmer, R. F., K. C. Lasseter: Sodiumnitroprusside. N. Engl. J. Med. **292** (1975) 294.

[10] Tillmanns, H.: Mikrozirkulation des Herzens. Habilitationsschrift, Heidelberg 1980.

Topical glyceryl trinitrate as adjunctive treatment in Raynaud's disease

A. G. Franks jr.

Introduction

Maurice Raynaud described the condition which bears his name in 1862 in a paper titled "On Local Asphyxia and Symmetrical Gangrene of the Extremeties." He reported an impressive array of clinical features describing peripheral vasomotor abnormalities which resulted in paroxysmal digital ischemia. In 1929, Thomas Lewis attempted to define the etiopathogenesis of these attacks, the study of which has continued to the present time, and remains poorly understood. Problems with terminology have caused difficulty in evaluating this group of patients, and lead to an International Symposium in Berlin in 1979, organized by the Cardiology Department of the Free University of Berlin in Cooperation with the German Society for Angiology, with Prof. Dr. Heinz Heidrich as symposium editor. The large number of therapeutic approaches, many without longterm clinical followup amplified the heterogeneous pathophysiology of the patients studied.

The treatment of Raynaud's disease remains unsatisfactory, especially in patients with an associated collagen disease. The effects of the various treatments are inconsistent, and their benefits are frequently not maintained. Abnormalities of both the central sympathetic nervous system and local digital vessels are implicated in the vasospasms, but the exact contributions of these, as well as other abnormalities, in each patient are not well understood. Since nitroglycerin can produce arterial, capillary and venular vasodilitation, and its local application has been studied since Lund's experiments in 1945 in the treatment of coronary artery disease, it seemed worth while to assess the clinical usefulness of commercially available glyceryl trinitrate ointment as a vasodilator in patients with Raynaud's disease.

Patient population and methods

In the trial there were 33 women and 4 men, aged 18–63 years, with bilateral Raynaud's disease diagnosed by the characteristic phasic colour changes, with or

Nitroglycerin 5

without pain, on exposure to cold. Patients had had symptoms for varying periods from 6 months to 10 years. All 37 patients had an associated collagen vascular disease: 13 patients had progressive systemic sclerosis (PSS); 23 patients had systemic lupus erythematosus (SLE); and 1 patient had rheumatoid arthritis (RA). All 13 patients with PSS were receiving either methyldopa (10 patients) or guanethidine (3 patients) at the maximum levels they could tolerate (methyldopa, 1–2 g/day; guanethidine, 10 mg/day) but still had persistent symptoms of Raynaud's disease. The drugs were maintained at the same levels for at least 1 month before and throughout the study. The 23 patients with SLE were either receiving oral prednisone, antimalarials, azathioprine, or NSAIDS for their primary disease, and the patient with RA was receiving aspirin. The levels of these drugs were also maintained throughout the study period. 1 patient with PSS had undergone bilateral cervical sympathectomy 3 years before the study. All patients were having at least one episode of bilateral vasospasm per week on entry to the study.

Glyceryl trinitrate 2% (Nitro-bid ointment, Marion Laboratories) was mixed with equal parts of lanolin to a final concentration of 1%. Initial trials with full strength (2%) preparations had been terminated owing to a high incidence of nitrate headache. The placebo preparation consisted of lanolin alone. Patients started with one preparation, and after 6 weeks each patient received the other preparation in a double-blind, crossover trial. The patients were instructed to apply the test preparation to one hand only; the opposite hand was used as an internal control to eliminate any effects of spontaneous remission. The preparations were applied by the patient to the digits only; a plastic glove was worn on the untreated hand. Preparations were applied three times daily and during acute vasospastic attacks. Patients applied an even, thin layer of the preparation without massaging or persistent rubbing; they were told that the total amount of each application should not exceed 4 inches (10 cm) measured by the dose measurement applicator supplied with active preparation. Each inch of medication contained approximately 8 mg of nitroglycerin. Therefore the total dose of nitroglycerin did not exceed approximately 35 mg of nitroglycerin. If headache occurred, the patient was instructed to reduce each following total dose.

Results

For all patients the trial took place during the cold weather months only. After initial assessment on entry to the study, patients were re-evaluated approximately every 2 weeks. Assessment was based upon frequency of attacks, severity of attacks, and the size of ulcers; patients were required to maintain a diary of both the frequency and severity of attacks. Frequency of attacks was rated on a scale of 1–4 as follows: 1. one per week or less; 2. more than one per week but less than one per day; 3. one per day; 4. more than one per day. Severity of attacks was rated on a scale of 1–3: 1. characteristic phasic colour change without numbness or pain; 2. colour change plus numbness; 3. colour change plus numbness and pain. The size of ulcers was estimated by a single observer who used the measurement of the largest diameter and recorded ulceration as improved, no change, or worse. The effects of the glyceryl trinitrate preparation and of the placebo on frequency and severity of attacks and size of ulcers were compared by the x-square analysis.

In comparison with placebo, glyceryl trinitrate ointment significantly reduced ($p < 0.001$) the frequency of attacks. 29 patients had fewer episodes of Raynaud's disease while using the active preparation, whereas only 8 patients had fewer attacks while using placebo. None of the patients had more frequent attacks during the glyceryl trinitrate period. Only 2 patients had more than three acute attacks per day and therefore applied ointment more frequently. One of these patients improved and the other did not. These data did not affect the x-square analysis.

Glyceryl trinitrate treatment also significantly reduced ($p < 0.001$) the severity of attacks. 25 patients had less associated numbness, pain, or both while using the active preparation, whereas only 1 patient noted improvement while on placebo. 2 patients had more severe attacks during the glyceryl trinitrate period, and 9 patients had more severe attacks during the placebo period.

12 patients had ulcerations during the study. The size of the ulcers was significantly reduced ($p < 0.005$) when patients were using the glyceryl trinitrate ointment. 10 of the 12 patients showed improvement in the size of ulcers during the glyceryl trinitrate period, whereas only 1 of the 12 showed improvement while using the placebo. None of the patients had more extensive ulceration during the glyceryl trinitrate period, whereas 5 of the 12 patients had more extensive ulceration while they were using the placebo.

Reduced capillary flow is the most important causative factor in Raynaud's disease, and the colour changes correlate well with the changes in capillary flow of the digit. The beneficial effects of glyceryl trinitrate are presumably due to vasodilatation with increased capillary flow to the digit. It was apparent during the study that glyceryl trinitrate also had systemic effects, since nitrate headache, postural hypotension, and abnormal sensations in the untreated hand were noted in a few patients. However, improvement occurred only in the treated hands, which suggests that it is the local effects of glyceryl trinitrate ointment which are important in Raynaud's disease.

Earlier studies on the use of glyceryl trinitrate in Raynaud's disease associated with collagen disease had disappointing results. However, all our patients with PSS were receiving the highest doses of methyldopa or guanethidine that they could tolerate; These drugs have been shown previously to have varying success in this disease. The glyceryl trinitrate was used as an adjunct to sympatholytic treatment in our patients. They were able to use the glyceryl trinitrate ointment during acute vasospastic attacks and reported substantially reduced symptoms in the treated digits. 2 of the patients who had required intra-arterial reserpine because of cyanosis and pain before the study were able to abort severe, acute vasospastic attacks with the glyceryl trinitrate 1% ointment; this treatment may be tried before such measures as intra-arterial reserpine injections are used.

Summary

The effects of topical glyceryl trinitrate in Raynaud's disease were compared with those of placebo in a double-blind, crossover trial in 37 patients with bilateral Raynaud's disease and an associated collagen disease, who were receiving oral sympatholytic agents at the maximum levels they could tolerate. 1% glyceryl trinitrate ointment or a placebo of lanolin was applied to one hand only for 6 weeks. The results were evaluated every 2 weeks. The frequency of attacks, severity of attacks, and size of ulcers in the treated hand were significantly lower when the patients were using glyceryl trinitrate ointment than when they were using placebo. The treatment of Raynaud's disease may be improved by using topical glyceryl trinitrate ointment as an adjunct to a basic regimen of oral sympatholytic agents. Glyceryl trinitrate ointment may obviate the need for more aggressive treatment, such as intra-arterial reserpine, in selected patients.

Supplementary reading

Coffman, J. D.: Vasodilator drugs in peripheral vascular disease. Engl. J. Med. **300** (1979) 713–717.

Coffman, J. D., A. S. Cohen: Total and capillary fingertip blood flow in Raynaud's phenomenon. N. Engl. J. Med. **285** (1971) 259–263.

Fischer, M., B. Reinhold, H. Falck et al.: Topical nitrolgycerin ointment in Raynaud's phenomenon. Z. Kardiol. **74** (1985) 298–302.

Franks jr., A. G.: Topical glyceryl trinitrate as adjunctive treatment in Raynaud's disease. Lancet **I** (1982) 76–77.

Halperin, J. L., J. D. Coffman: Patholphysiology of Raynaud's disease. Arch. Intern. Med. **139** (1979) 89–92.

Heidrich, H. (eds.): Raynaud's Phenomenon. International Symposium of the Angiologic Working Group and Cardiology Department of the Medical Clinics of the Free University of Berlin, Clinicum Charlottenburg, in Cooperation with the German Society for Angiology. TM-Verlag, Berlin 1979.

Kleckner, M. S., E. V. Allen, G. W. Khalil: The effect of local application of glyceryl trinitrate (nitroglycerin) on Raynaud's disease and Raynaud's phenomenon. Circulation **3** (1951) 681–689.

Kleckner, M. S., E. V. Allen, K. G. Wakim: The use of glyceryl trinitrate in the treatment of Raynaud's phenomenon. Proc. Staff. Meet., Mayo Clin. **25** (1960) 657–658.

Kontos, H. A., A. J. Wasserman: Effect of reserpine in Raynaud's phenomenon. Circulation **39** (1969) 259–266.

LeRoy, E. C., J. A. Downey, P. J. Cannon: Skin capillary blood flow scleroderma. J. Clin. Invest. **50** (1971) 930–939.

Lund, F.: Administration of nitroglycerin through the skin and ulcer surfaces. Nord. Med. **29** (1946) 194.

Lund, F.: Percutaneous nitroglycerin treatment in cases of peripheral circulatory disorders, especially Raynaud's disease. Acta Med. Scand. (suppl. 206) **130** (1948) 196.

Thomas, M., H. Campbell, G. Heard: The effect of vasodilator drugs on skin blood flow in peripheral vascular occlusion. Br. J. Surg. **55** (1968) 588–590.

Varadi, D. P., A. M. Lawrence: Suppression of Raynaud's phenomenon by methyldopa. Arch. Intern. Med. **124** (1969) 13–18.

Studies of glyceryl trinitrate application in gastroenterology

M. Staritz, K.-H. Meyer zum Büschenfelde

Part I The dilative effect on the bile duct sphincter (sphincter of Oddi) and endoscopic extraction of bile duct calculi through the intact sphincter

The sphincter of Oddi is the duodeno-biliary junction. Tonus and motility of its smooth muscle have the physiological function of regulating bile and pancreas flow and of preventing duodeno-biliary reflux. However, this sphincter is an obstacle to endoscopic extraction of biliary calculi. For this reason it was usually destroyed through endoscopic papillosphincterotomy. This method carries a rate of complications of around 8% and a lethality rate of 1.2% [4].

Glyceryl trinitrate is known for its dilative effect on smooth muscle. It has been in use for a long time for instance in angiology and for treating coronary heart disease. Since the sphincter of Oddi is made up of smooth muscle, we studied the effect of glyceryl trinitrate on its basal tonus and sphincter contractions.

In the present paper it is demonstrated that nitroglycerin (glyceryl trinitrate) results in medicinal sphincter dilation. This effect enables an endoscopic extraction of bile duct calculi to be made through the intact papilla without endoscopic papillosphincterotomy which would otherwise be required.

Methodology

Analysing the effect of glyceryl trinitrate on the sphincter of Oddi (ERCP-manometry)

ERCP manometry was performed before retrograde cholangiography in 17 patients who underwent endoscopic retrograde cholangiopancreaticography in order to rule out a pancreticobiliary disease. In all patients gastric and duodenal ulcers, diabetes mellitus, systemic diseases as well as alcoholism had been excluded. There was no

Nitroglycerin 5

case of medication with a potential influence on gastro-intestinal motility. All patients were informed about the study and had given their consent. They were subdivided into two groups:

"Nitro group"
In 9 patients (5 men, 4 women, mean age 43 years) before and 3 minutes after applying 1.2 mg of glyceryl trinitrate (Nitrolingual-Spray®, Pohl-Boskamp, Hohenlockstedt) the basal tonus of the sphincter of Oddi, its rate and amplitude of contraction were determined.

Control group
The corresponding manometric examination was furthermore made in 8 patients (5 men, 3 women, mean age 40 years) without administering glyceryl trinitrate.

Endoscopic manometry

After a 12-hour fasting period and premedication with 10–15 mg of diazepam (i.v.) which does not have any influence on the sphincter of Oddi's motility [1] the ERCP manometry was performed. To this end the sphincter of Oddi was cannulated with a three-lumen capillary catheter of 1.6 mm outer diameter using the standard ERCP technique (Olympus JF 1 T endoscope). Two of the capillaries are perfused with physiological saline (0.1 ml per minute) and each of these is linked with a pressure transducer (Statham element, Beckman R 427 G). The capillaries end in side-openings in the region of the catheter tip.

The manometric investigation always starts by determining the duodenal pressure; then the pressure of the bile duct is determined and finally the sphincter of Oddi's motility and its basal pressure is investigated.

When evaluating the measurement tracing shown schematically in figure I-1, the duodenal pressure is the reference point for determining the other pressure levels.

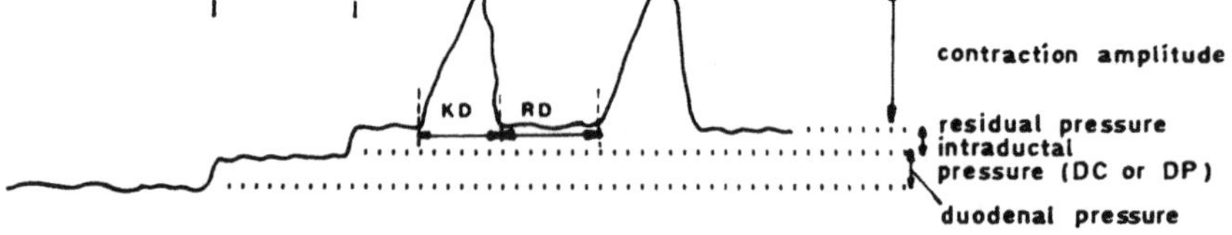

Fig. I-1 Typical behaviour of the pressure curve for endoscopic manometry in the duodenum, ductus choledochus and sphincter of Oddi.

The contraction amplitude of the papilla is measured against the level of its basal tonus [1, 2, 7, 8].

Results

The basal tonus of the sphincter of Oddi, its rate and amplitude of contraction were comparable in the "nitro group" and in the control group (fig. I-1). The administration of glyceryl trinitrate reduced the sphincter of Oddi's basal pressure from 8.8 ± 0.7 mmHg to 2.6 ± 0.9 mmHg ($p < 0.005$). The rate of contraction was not influenced by glyceryl trinitrate.

In the control group no difference in results was found between the first and the second measurement (fig. I-2).

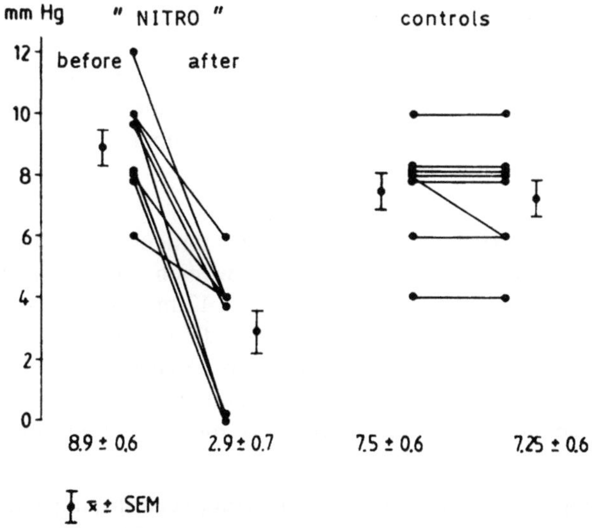

Fig. I-2 Influence of glyceryl trinitrate (1.2 mg sublingually) on the basal tonus of the sphincter of Oddi.

Endoscopic extraction of bile duct stones through the glyceryl trinitrate-dilated papilla

Method

Diagnostic endoscopy

The standard technique was used for the endoscopic retrograde cholangio-pancreaticography (Olympus JF 1 T endoscope, Rayvist 300 contrast medium, Schering AG, Frankfurt). For premedication we gave 10–15 mg of diazepam and 40 mg of N-butyl scopolamine. In order to determine what size the bile duct stones were we used the known diameter of the endoscope as a reference represented in the radiographs [8].

Therapeutic endoscopy

For medicinal dilation of the sphincter of Oddi 1.2 mg of glyceryl trinitrate (Nitrolingual-Spray®, Pohl-Boskamp, Hohenlockstedt) were administered. 2–3 minutes later the sphincter of Oddi was intubated with a large diameter dormia basked (Olympus FG 16 L, 2.2 mm diameter). The dilative action of glyceryl trinitrate was considered to be sufficient if this dormia probe could be introduced spontaneously into the bile duct through the papilla. When this was not possible, up to two times 1.2 mg of glyceryl trinitrate was given at 2–3 minute intervals. Nevertheless the papilla could not be intubated in 4 patients.

After intubation of the bile duct the concrements were caught with the dormia basket and extracted under endoscopic view (figs. I-3 a–c). If this was not possible, the dormia basket and therefore the papilla were pulled up close to the tip of the endoscope and the concrement was extracted by pulling the endoscope itself. If the patient had complaints as a result, we used mechanical lithotripsy. (lithotriptor: prototype, Wolf company or Erlangen lithotriptor, Wolf company, Knittlingen).

Results

The described procedure was tried on 25 patients. In 4 patients intubation of the papilla did not succeed. The remaining 21 (6 men, 15 women, mean age 58 years) had a total of 32 bile duct stones with a diameter of 6–12 mm removed. 5 of the patients had residual stones following immediately preceding cholecystectomy. In 9 patients cholecystectomy had been performed 1–12 years ago and 3 patients had not been cholecystectomised but did not have any other choleliths. In these patients 32 calculi were extracted spontaneously. In 4 patients mechanical lithotripsy was required for concrements of 9–12 mm diameter.

During and after endoscopic removal of the calculi no complications, in particular no pancreatitis nor any cholangitis occurred, with the exception of a temporary headache (14 patients) induced by nitroglycerin administration.

For all patients a control ERCP was carried out after 3 to 8 days. In one female patient we found a concrement of 8 mm diameter which had previously been overlooked and could now be removed. In all the persons examined the papilla was without pathological findings endoscopically and radiologically and continued to be competent. A follow-up examination performed on 6 patients by means of ERCP manometry did not reveal any change in their motility parameters and in residual papillary pressure.

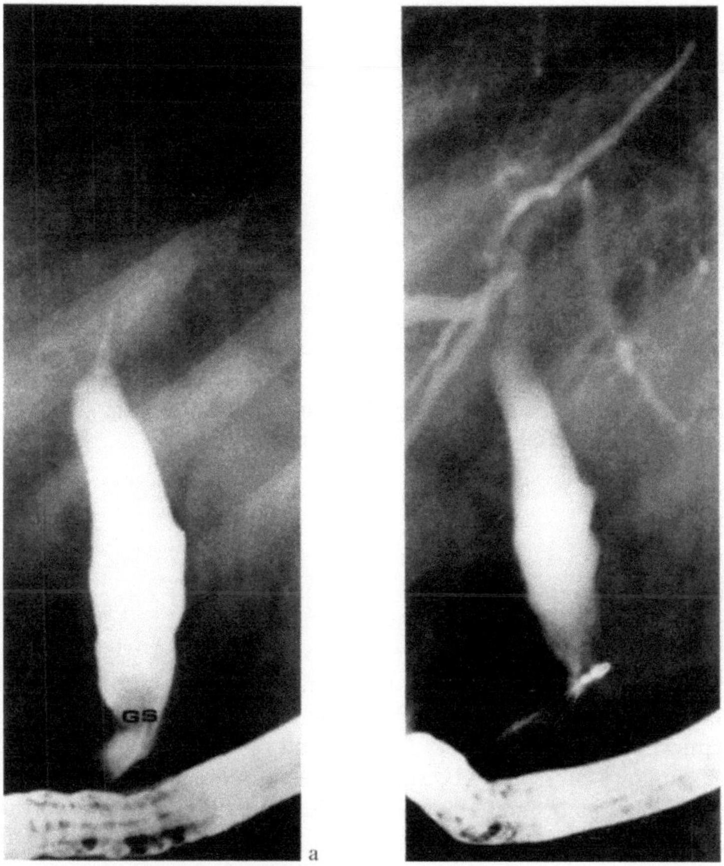

a b

Fig. I-3a Small choledochus concrement (GS).
Fig. I-3b Choledochus concrement caugt in the dormia basket.

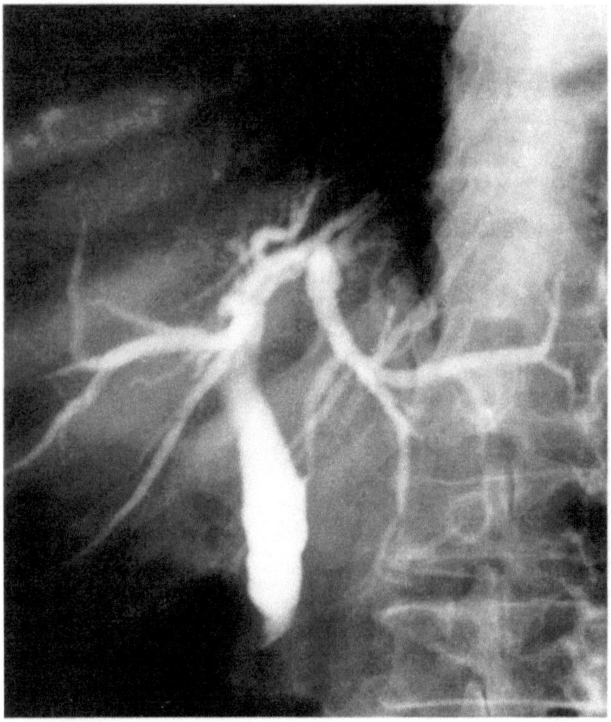

c

Fig. I-3c Stoneless biliary duct after extraction of the choledochus concrement, after "drug induced papillary dilatation" following administration of 1.2 mg glyceryl trinitrate. The papilla is also competent after stone extraction.

Discussion

Through ERCP manometry it could be shown that glyceryl trinitrate causes the smooth muscle of the sphincter of Oddi to relax. A previous pilot study of our own demonstrated that N-butyl scopolaminebromide at the dosage used here leads to a total interruption of papillary motility for a period of 4–6 minutes while it does not reduce basal papillary pressure. The simultaneous application of glyceryl trinitrate and N-butyl scopolaminebromide induces the described dilative effect in the papilla and an interruption of its contractions.

The endoscopic extraction of small and medium-sized bile duct stones through the intact papilla dilated temporarily by nitroglycerin was easy to do in technical terms.

No complications occurred. A risk to the patient could be excluded by applying mechanical lithotripsy which was developed by Demling et al. [3] and is always a success, in particular for small and medium-sized concretions. A follow-up of the treated patients showed that sphincter function was not impaired due to the performed endoscopic manipulation.

The described method, enabled through the dilative effect of glyceryl trinitrate on the sphincter of Oddi allows a large percentage of patients with choledocholithiasis to be treated without the relatively risky endoscopic papillotomy common up to now. A recently developed alternative to this invasive endoscopic procedure is endoscopic dilation of the sphincter muscle by means of a special balloon catheter [5]. Since this method is expensive because of the high price of the balloon catheter, "medical papillary dilation", means a considerable reduction of treatment costs.

In addition to what we believe is an impressive new field of application of glyceryl trinitrate we were able to find in clinical routine that when carrying out retrograde cholangiopancreaticography the sublingual application of glyceryl trinitrate (1.2 mg of nitrolingual spray) enabled the bile duct and the pancreatic duct to be intubated in most cases when the experienced endoscopist had not succeeded in doing so spontaneously. In this way without further manipulations of the sphincter muscle endoscopic measures such as transpapillary forceps biopsy from the bile duct became possible and moreover therapeutic procedures could be performed which usually can only be done after papillotomy, such as placing a transpapillary endoprosthesis.

Our study results suggest that nitroglycerin (glyceryl trinitrate) might act as a spasmolytic in the region of smooth muscles of the biliary tract and the sphincter of Oddi. Whether this expectation is met can only be revealed by further studies.

References

[1] Nebel, O. T.: Manometric evaluation of the papilla of Vater. Gastroenterol. Endosc. **21** (1975) 126–128.

[2] Arndorfer, R. C., J. J. Steff, W. J. Dodds et al.: Improved infusion system for intraluminal oesophageal manometry. Gastroenterology **24** (1977) 7–23.

[3] Demling, L., K. Seuberth, J. F. Riemann: A mechanical lithotripter. Endoscopy **14** (1982) 100–101.

[4] Seifert, E., K. Gail, J. Weismüller: Langzeitresultate nach endoskopischer Sphinkterotomie. Dtsch. Med. Wochenschr. **107** (1982) 610–616.

[5] Staritz, M., K. Ewe, K.-H. Meyer zum Büschenfelde: Endoscopic papillary dilation (EPD) for the treatment of common bile duct stones and papillary stenosis. Endoscopy **15** (1983) 197–198.

[6] Staritz, M., T. Poralla, K. Ewe et al.: Effect of glyceryl trinitrate on the sphincter of Oddi motility and baseline pressure. Gut **26** (1985) 194–197.

[7] Staritz, M., K. Ewe, K.-H. Meyer zum Büschenfelde: Die endoskopische Papillen- und Gallenwegsmanometrie zur Funktionsdiagnostik der Papilla Vateri. Untersuchungen bei Patientinnen mit Cholezystolithiasis. Schweiz. Rundschau Med. (PRAXIS) **73** (1984) 1287–1289.
[8] Staritz, M., T. Poralla, K. Klose et al.: The endoscope – a reliable parameter for assessment of the diameter of the bile duct and bile duct stones. Z. Gastroenterol. **22** (1984) 697–700.

Part II The influence on the intravascular oesophageal variceal pressure (IOVP) in patients suffering from cirrhosis of the liver

Bleeding of oesophageal varices always is a life-threatening situation to the patient with cirrhosis of the liver. First reports by Lebrec [8] gave rise to the hope that his complication could be controlled medicinally. Since further studies [3, 10] suggested that the beta receptor blockers first used were inappropriate, the search for other substances started.

The dilative action of glyceryl trinitrate on vascular muscle is well documented. While Freeman and Groszman [5, 6] observed a favourable influence in a clinical setting, Dawson and Hallemans [4, 7] did not find the expected influence when studying isosorbite dinitrate.

We developed a method recently permitting a direct determination of blood pressure to be made in the oesophageal varices, that is at the site of bleeding [13]. This method was used to investigate the influence of glyceryl trinitrate whose rapid onset of action and short half life are well-known [14].

Method

Patients

16 patients (9 men, 7 women, from 40 to 63 years old, mean age 54 years) with histologically established hepatic cirrhosis (Child A) were investigated. All patients had had at least one incident of bleeding oesophageal varices as verified by endoscopy. 4 of these patients were under spironolactone treatment (50 mg a day). The taking of beta receptor blockers or other durgs having a potential effect on portal hypertension was ruled out.

Endoscopic determination of oesophageal variceal pressure

Oesophagoscopy was performed on these patients with a flexible endoscope (Olympus GIF-Q). The oesophageal varices were classified according to Paquet [11] into medium-sized varices grade II (n = 6) and very large varices grade III (n = 10).

Pressure measurement was made by puncturing the oesophageal varices with a fine needle (sclerosing needle, outside diameter 0.71 mm) which was perfused with physiological saline (0.2 ml per minute) by means of a hydraulic capillary pump [1] and connected to a Statham element (Beckman R 427 G). Each investigation started with a determination of the oesophageal pressure by positioning the fine needle within the oesophageal lumen. The difference between the pressure prevailing in the oesophagos and the varicees is called intravascular oesophageal variceal pressure (IOVP) (fig. II-1).

The action of glyceryl trinitrate was determined by measuring IOVP before and 3 minutes after the sublingual administration of 1.2 mg of glyceryl trinitrate (Nitrolingual-Spray®, Pohl-Boskamp, Hohenlockstedt).

All levels are expressed as a mean ($\bar{x}$) ± SEM. A statistical analysis of pressure levels before and after giving glyceryl trinitrate was made with the combined Wilcoxon test.

Results

The IOVP in grade II varices was 16.3 ± 0.4 mmHg and in grade III varices 22.8 ± 2 mmHg (fig. II-2). Three minutes after administering 1.2 mg of glyceryl trinitrate the IOVP dropped sharply in all patients without any exception (fig. II-3). In relation to the size of these oesophageal varices this means that the IOVP in grade III varices was reduced to 10 ± 0.4 mmHg and in grade III varices to 12 ± 0.4 mmHg (fig. II-2).

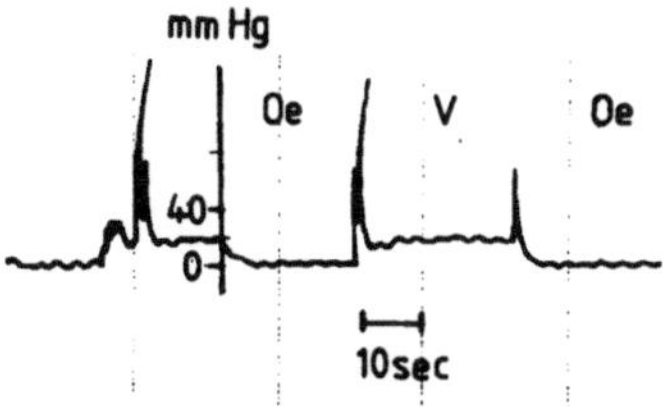

Fig. II-1 Example of a tracing to determine the intravascular oesophageal variceal pressure (IOVP). The IOVP is measured as the pressure difference between the oesophageal diameter and the variceal diameter (V).

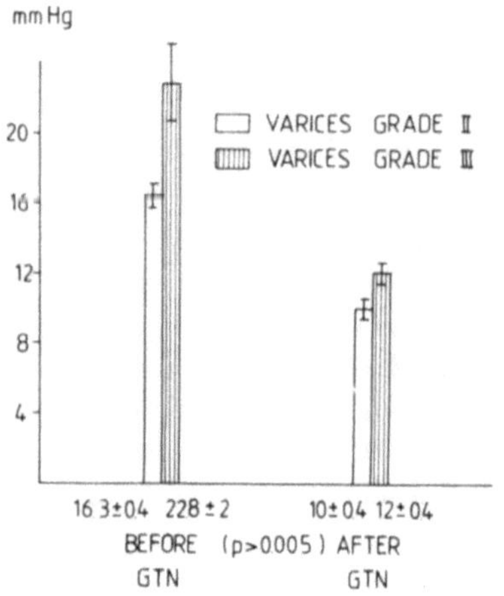

Fig. II-2 Action of glyceryl trinitrate (GTN) on IOVP (n = 16).

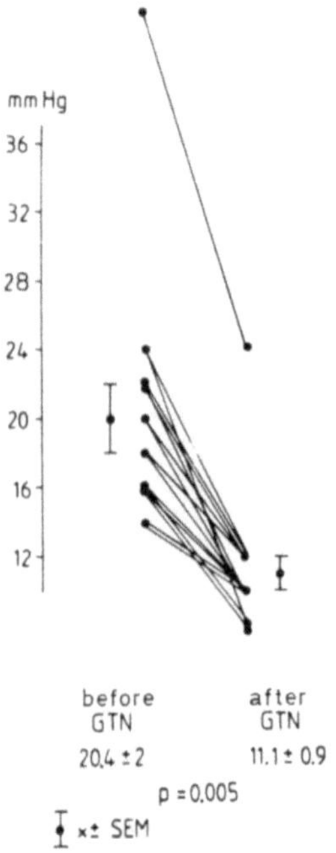

Fig. II-3 Action of glyceryl trinitrate (GTN) on IOVP in grade II varices (n = 6) and grade III varices (n = 10).

In none of the investigated patients was there any complication to be attributed to the endoscopic determination of the IOVP. Inasmuch as there was a slight oozing haemorrhage from the puncture site, this could be compressed in all cases by advancing the endoscope forward into the stomach for about 3 minutes.

Discussion

The endoscopic method presented to determine the intravascular oesophageal variceal pressure proved to be easy to carry out, safe to apply and appropriate for studying the influence of a drug on the IOVP. In our view this pressure is of greater importance to the risk of bleeding than the indirect methods known up to now for determining portal pressure and hepatic vein pressure [2, 19].

To date no other drug was shown to lower IOVP. Glyceryl trinitrate therefore seems to be appropriate at this time to the treatment of bleeding oesophageal varices. When treating such patients with glyceryl trinitrate (5 mg an hour i.v.) we observed correspondingly favourable therapeutic successes. Compared with vasoconstrictors (e.g. vasopressin) glyceryl trinitrate has the advantage of easy control. Moreover it avoids typical adverse reactions found with vasoconstrictors such as ischaemia of the myocardium.

There cannot be any doubt that further investigations are needed in order to clarify the ideal dosage in applying glyceryl trinitrate and to find the requisite duration of application, not least with respect to potential tolerance effects. The question of whether nitrobodies might assume importance in preventing variceal bleeding must be answered by further studies.

References

[1] Arndorfer, R. C., J. J. Steff, W. J. Dodds et al.: Improved infusion system for intraluminal oesophageal manometry. Gastroenterology **72** (1977) 7–23.

[2] Boyer, T. D., D. R. Triger, M. Horisawa et al.: Direct transhepatic measurement of portal vein pressure using a thin needle. Gastroenterology **72** (1977) 584–589.

[3] Burroughs, A. K., W. J. Jenkins, S. Sherlock: Controlled trial of propranolol for the prevention of recurrent variceal hemorrhage in patients with cirrhosis. N. Engl. J. Med. **309** (1983) 1539–1542.

[4] Dawson, J., R. West, P. Gertsch et al.: Endoscopic variceal pressure measurements: Response to isosorbite dinitrate. Gut **24** (1983) A 971.

[5] Freeman, J. G., J. R. Barton, D. D. Record: Effects of vasodilators on portal pressure in patients with portal hypertension. Gut **24** (1983) A 971.

[6] Groszman, R. J., D. Kravetz, J. Bosch: Nitroglycerin improves the hemodynamic response to vasopressin in portal hypertension. Hepatology **2** (1982) 757–762.
[7] Hallemans, R., R. Naeije, P. Mols et al.: Treatment of portal hypertension with isosorbite dinitrate alone and in combination with vasopressin. Crit. Care Med. **11** (1983) 536–540.
[8] Lebrec, D., T. Poynard, P. Hillon et al.: Propranolol for prevention of recurrent gastrointestinal bleeding in patients with cirrhosis. N. Engl. J. Med. **305** (1981) 1371–1374.
[9] McLeod, M. K., F. E. Eckhauser, J. G. Turcotte: Significance of corrected sinusoidal pressure (CSP) in patients with cirrhosis and portal hypertension. Ann. Surg. **194** (1981) 562–567.
[10] Mills, P. R., A. P. Rae, D. A. Farah et al.: Comparison of three adrenoreceptor blocking agents in patients with cirrhosis and postal hypertension. Gut **25** (1984) 73–78.
[11] Paquet, K. J.: Prophylactic endoscopic sclerosing treatment of the oesophageal wall in varices – A prospective controlled randomized trial. Endoscopy **14** (1982) 4–5.
[12] Rose, J. D. R., M. D. Crane, P. M. Smith: Factors affecting successful endoscopic sclerotherapy for oesophageal varices. Gut **24** (1983) 946–949.
[13] Staritz, M., T. Poralla, K.-H. Meyer zum Büschenfelde: Intravascular oesophageal variceal pressure (IOVP) assessed by endoscopic fine needle puncture under basal conditions, Valsalva's manoeuvre and after glyceryltrinitrate application. Gut **26** (1985) 525-530.
[14] Armstrong, P. W., J. A. Armstrong, G. S. Marks: Blood levels after sublingual nitroglycerin. Circulation **59** (1979) 585–588.

Regional ventricular function before and after sublingual nitroglycerin in patients with a recent myocardial infarction, during the subacute and chronic phase

W.-D. Bussmann, H. Sievert, R. Geiß, F. D. Maul, M. Kaltenbach

Introduction

The results of numerous clinical and experimental investigations indicate that a myocardial infarction usually reaches its final dimensions within a few hours of its onset. On the other hand it is known that vital but ischaemic myocardium remains at the periphery of the infarcted area. It is not yet clear whether this ischeamic myocardium remains ischaemic, gradually becomes necrotic and thus – clinically unnoticed – increases the size of the infarct, or whether it is well supplied with blood and capable of normal functioning again after the formation of collaterals or recanalization of the primarily occluded vessel.

We investigated the global and regional ventricular function of 7 patients at the subacute (third/fourth day) and chronic (third week) phase of infarction. To permit differentiation between disturbed ventricular function resulting from ischaemia and that caused by a scar, the investigation was in all cases conducted before and after administration of nitroglycerin.

Patients and method

The investigation comprised 7 patients with a myocardial infarction verified clinically, by electrocardiograph and by enzymatic analysis. The mean age was 52 +/− 5 years. Six of the patients had the infarct in the anterior wall and 1 patient in the posterior wall. All the patients were first examined on the third or fourth day and then again after three weeks. The pulmonary capillary pressure measured in 6 patients as an indication of left-ventricular filling pressure was 7–12 mmHg in 4 cases and increased to above 15 mmHg in the other two.

Prior to and 3–5 minutes after sublingual administration of 1.6 mg nitroglycerin (Nitrolingual®, Pohl-Boskamp), an ECG-triggered heart chamber scintigraphy was

Nitroglycerin 5

carried out in left anterior oblique projection [6, 8, 9, 11, 12] with 99 m Technetium. In addition to the global ejection fraction the regional ejection fraction was also determined in 9 equiangular section and the result stated as a percentage of the normal value for each sector (relative percent [11]). The segment with the relatively lowest ejection fraction (EF) was termed the infarcted segment and that with the highest EF the non-infarcted segment.

The analysis for statistical significance was made by the t-test for paired samples. In each case the mean and the standard error of the mean (SEM) were stated.

Results

During the subacute phase of the infarction the global EF was lowered to an average of 31 +/− 4%, and after three weeks to 37 +/− 6%. The slight rise was not significant ($p > 0.05$) (fig. 1). On the 3rd/4th day the regional EF in the infarcted area was 22 +/− 9 relative percent. Three weeks later it had in all cases increased, the average being 38 +/− 11 relative percent ($p < 0.05$). The regional EF in the non-infarcted segment did not alter significantly (on average, an increase from 74 +/− 5 to 85 +/− 13 relative percent).

During the subacute phase of infarction the global EF did not alter significantly after administration of nitroglycerin, the average rise being from 31 +/− 4 to 34 +/− 5% ($p > 0.05$) (fig. 1). The regional EF in the infarcted area increased in all cases after nitroglycerin and rose from a mean of 22 +/− 9 to 35 +/− 11 relative percent ($p < 0.05$) (fig. 2). In the non-infarcted segment nitroclycerin did not induce a significant change in the regional EF – a mean rise from 74 +/− 5 to 77 +/− 7 relative percent ($p > 0.05$).

Three weeks after infarction the administration of nitroglycerin did not result in a significant change in the EF. In the mean the global EF rose from 37 +/− 6 to 40 +/ − 6% ($p > 0.05$); the regional EF in the infarcted segment increased from 38 +/− 11 to 48 +/− 11 relative percent ($p > 0.05$) and the regional EF in the non-infarcted segment rose from 85 +/− 13 to 90 +/− 11 relative percent ($p > 0.05$).

Discussion

The ischaemia tolerance of the myocardium is relatively brief. After acute occlusion of a coronary vessel the ensuing myocardial infarction often reaches its virtually final extent within a few hours. At the periphery of the infarct, especially in the

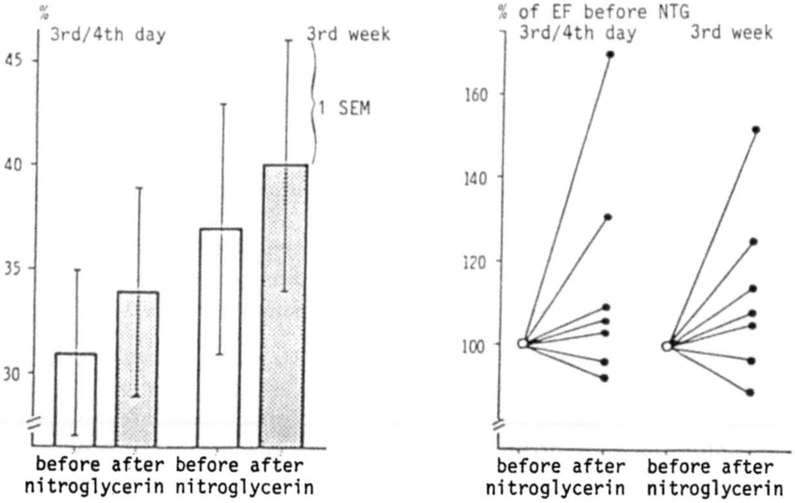

Fig. 1 Global ejection fraction before and after sublingual administration of 1.6 mg nitroglycerin in recent myocardial infarction. Both in the subacute phase of the infarction (3rd/4th day) and at the chronic stage (3rd week) an improvement in ventricular function was observed after administration of nitroglycerin (n = 7).

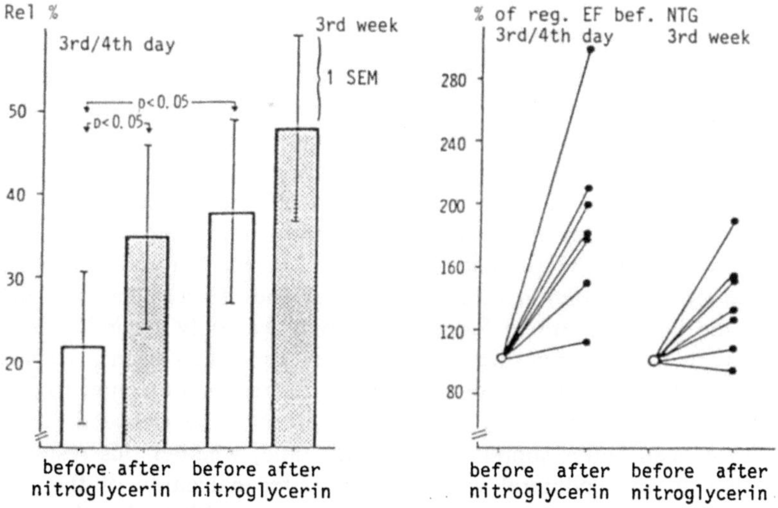

Fig. 2 Regional ejection fraction in the infarcted area before and after sublingual administration of 1.6 mg nitroglycerin. The improvement in functional activity occurring during the healing process from the 3rd/4th day to the 3rd week corresponds in extent to the improvement achieved with nitroglycerin on 3rd/4th day (n = 7).

epicardium, ischaemic myocardium may however persist, and little is known about its fate. It is possible that this ischaemic area returns completely to normal after the formation of collaterals or recanalization of the coronary vessel in which occlusion occurred; but it is just as possible that cells are gradually destroyed, thus increasing the size of the infarct.

Both ischaemia and myocardial necrosis result in an impairment of function in the area concerned. The functioning of ischaemic myocardium can however be influenced, at least in part [10], by administration of nitroglycerin. Improved functioning after nitroglycerin in a specific area of the myocardium suggests that such improvement may also be expected after establishment of an aortocoronary bypass [5].

In all the patients investigated there was an improvement in regional ventricular function in the infarcted area following administration of nitroglycerin 3–4 days after the infarction. This was also true of patients with normal filling pressure. Evidently none of the patients suffered from reduced perfusion of the infarcted area as a result of a fall in arterial blood pressure.

Other authors have also reported a very definite improvement in functional activity in the infarcted segment when nitroglycerin was given in the first few days [7]. This may be interpreted as a sign of ischaemia at rest persisting after the infarction, and tends to indicate the presence of vital myocardium. Three weeks after the infarction, on the other hand, no substantial improvement in functional activity could be detected after administration of nitroglycerin.

In the subacute phase, regional functional activity in the infarcted segment is severely impaired, with an EF of 22 relative percent. In general, improved functioning of the infarcted segment is not to be expected during the first 3–4 days [1]. After administration of nitroglycerin at the subacute stage there was a very considerable functional improvement of about 90%. Obviously nitroglycerin makes it possible to influence the existing dysfunction – probably by improving the regional blood supply due to reduction in preload or dilatation of the coronary vessels. After consolidation of the infarction three weeks later the effect of nitroglycerin was lessened as the improvement in functional activity was only around 40%. In the interval between the two investigations, however, there had been a considerable improvement in function in the infarcted area. The regional ejection fraction had increased accordingly from 22 to 38 relative percent. The ischaemic area must therefore have been better supplied during this time, whether this resulted from improved flow in the collateral vessels or from recanalization of the primarily occluded vessel that caused the infarction. It seems more likely that the maximum improvement in function that can be achieved after three weeks is determined during the acute phase. The extent of the ischaemic myocardium, still capable of functioning, that can be "revealed" by nitroglycerin corresponds to the improvement that can be recorded after three weeks. Normally the regional EF during the subacute phase of infarction is 22 relative percent. After nitroglycerin it rises to 35 relative percent and reaches 38 relative percent in the course of the chronic phase. Three weeks after the infarction, sensitivity to nitroglycerin is reduced as the ischaemic myocardium has regained its ability to function.

Treatment with nitrates in cases of recent myocardial infarction seems to lead to a considerable improvement in functional activity in the infarcted segment, also in the subacute stage (3rd/4th day). It remains uncertain whether the improvement brought about by nitroglycerin is the result of a direct increase in blood supply – as for example through the opening of collaterals or dilatation of stenosis. Another possibility is an indirect increase in perfusion through a reduction of filling pressure. It is interesting that the improvement in function achieved in the infarcted area after nitroglycerin at the subacute stage corresponds approximately to the condition attained in the chronic phase after three weeks through spontaneous consolidation in the infarcted area [4]. Thereafter nitroglycerin is not able to induce an important increase in contractility in the infarcted area. If any recommendations for treatment can be drawn from these findings it would seem appropriate to follow up parenteral administration of nitroglycerin at the acute stage [2, 3] with nitrate treatment in oral form.

Summary

Seven patients with a recent myocardial infarction and mostly normal left ventricular end-diastolic pressure were investigated by radionuclide ventriculography after 3/4 days and three weeks before and after 1.6 mg nitroglycerin.

Between day 3/4 and the third week global ejection fraction rose unimportantly and insignificantly ($p > 0.05$) from 31 +/− 4 to 37 +/− 6 percent. The regional ejection fraction in the not infarcted area remained nearly stable (74 +/− 5 to 85 +/− 13 relative percent, $p > 0.05$). However, the ejection fraction in the infarcted area rose from 22 +/− 9 to 38 +/− 11 relative percent ($p < 0.05$ percent). On day 3/4 nitroglycerin induced a clear increase of the ejection fraction in the infarcted area from 22 +/− 9 to 35 +/− 11 relative percent ($p < 0.05$). The ejection fraction global and in the not infarcted area remained nearly constant (global EF from 31 +/− 4 to 34 +/− 5 percent, EF in the not infarcted area from 74 +/− 5 to 77 +/− 7 relative percent; $p > 0.05$). Three weeks after the myocardial infarction 1.6 mg nitroglycerin did not produce a significant alteration of the ejection fraction (slight increase of the global EF from 37 +/− 6 to 40 +/− 6, the regional EF in the infarcted area from 38 +/− 11 to 48 +/− 11 relative percent and from 85 +/− 13 to 90 +/− 11 relative percent in the not infarcted area; $p > 0.05$).

Obviously the relative high dosis of 1.6 mg nitroglycerin sublingual does not cause a depression of myocardial function in the infarcted area – even in patients with normal left ventricular end-diastolic pressure. The increase in the regional contractility after nitroglycerin equals the increase in the following three weeks. It may be, that there is vital ischemic myocardium in the infarcted area, which consolidates between the third and the 21st day and becomes insensitive to nitroglycerin.

This favorable effect of nitroglycerin may be the consequence of dilatation of coronary artery stenosis or opening of collateral vessels. Also an indirect effect and lowering of the left ventricular filling pressure is possible. These results support the continuation of the nitrate therapy beyond the acute phase of myocardial infarction.

References

[1] Bussmann, W.-D.: Akuter Myokardinfarkt. Klinik, Hämodynamik und nuklearmedizinische Untersuchungen. Therapiewoche **32** (1982) 6309.

[2] Bussmann, W.-D., D. Passek, W. Seidel et al.: Reduction of CK and CKMB indices of infarct size by intravenous nitroglycerin. Circulation **63** (1981) 615.

[3] Bussmann, W.-D., H. Schöfer, H. Kurita et al.: Nitroglycerin in acute myocardial infarction. X. Effect of small and large doses of nitroglycerin on sigma ST segment deviation – experimental and clinical results. Clin. Cardiol. **2** (1979) 106.

[4] Dunn, R. F., E. H. Botvinick, W. Benge et al.: The significance of nitroglycerin-induced changes in ventricular function after acute myocardial infarction. Am. J. Cardiol. **49** (1982) 1719.

[5] Helfant, R. H., R. Pine, S. G. Meister et al.: Nitroglycerin to unmask reversible asynergy. Correlation with postcoronary-bypass ventriculography. Circulation **50** (1974) 108.

[6] Maul, F. D., R. Standke, G. Hör: Nuklearmedizinische Diagnostik des akuten Myokardinfarktes. Therapiewoche **32** (1982) 6322.

[7] Ramanathan, K., M. M. Bodenheimer, V. S. Banka et al.: Natural history of contractile abnormalities after acute myocardial infarction in man: Severity and response to nitroglycerin as a function of time. Circulation **63** (1981) 731.

[8] Rigo, P., M. Murray, H. W. Strauss et al.: Left ventricular function in acute myocardial infarction, evaluated by gated scintiphotography. Circulation **50** (1974) 678.

[9] Sauer, E., H. Sebening, G. Hör et al.: Nichtinvasive Erfassung der Dynamik des linken Ventrikels. Bestimmung der linksventrikulären Auswurffraktion, der Ventrikelvolumina und der regionalen Wandbewegung durch die EKG-getriggerte Herzbinnenraumszintigraphie. Dtsch. Med. Wochenschr. **103** (1978) 1199.

[10] Schneider, W., S. Kohl, B. Kunkel et al.: Untersuchungen zur Reversibilität akinetischer Segmente bei der koronaren Herzkrankheit. Z. Kardiol. **73** (1984) 568.

[11] Standke, R., G. Hör, F. D. Maul: Ventrikel- und Myokardszintigraphie. Methodische Grundlagen. Therapiewoche **32** (1982) 6330.

[12] Wynne, J., M. Sayres, D. E. Maddox et al.: Regional left ventricular function in acute myocardial infarction: evaluation with quantitative radionuclide ventriculography. Am. J. Cardiol. **45** (1980) 203.

Therapy of coronary heart disease with nitrates in combination with other antianginal agents

M. Stauch

The treatment of angina pectoris is based on different classes of drugs with different pharmakodynamic profile: Venous vasodilators reduce preload, betablockers attenuate contractility and heart rate and calcium entry blockers act as arterial vasodilators. Calcium entry blockers may be subdivided into a more vasoactive (nifedipine) and a myocardial type (verapamil). They all reduce oxygen demand as main mechanism of antianginal action.

Frequently, a combination of drugs is used today for the treatment of angina. Mostly, venous vasodilators such as nitrates and molsidomine are combined with betablockers or calcium entry blockers. Since betablockers do not combine favorably with some calcium entry blockers, the combination of these two is relatively seldom used. Still, positive interaction on ischemic regions was also reported, e.g. for acebutolol and nifedipine [9].

For reasons of "myocardial protection" and certain prophylactic indications these classes of drugs are widely used beyond the indication angina pectoris. The extended indication comprises patients with chronic infarction without typical angina. These patients present with varying degrees of left ventricular impairment. Treatment with these drugs may have positive and with some of them potentially negative effects on global left ventricular function. This depends on the size and distribution of areas of myocardium of different disease states: 1. myocardium perfused by normal coronary arteries, 2. myocardium perfused by stenotic or collateral coronary arteries, exhibiting more or less severe signs of ischemia, when oxygen demand is increased and 3. scar tissue, which a) may not be transmural in extent and b) may have varying degrees of distensibility (dyskinesia), important for the effect of preload-reducing drugs. The use of combinations of drugs may reduce negative effects of a single drug by positive interactions. Negative interactions must also be considered.

Earlier, we have examined the effect of ISDN alone [12, 13] and the combination of the betablocker metoprolol and ISDN with radionuclideventriculography (RNV) combined with thermodilution technique for the measurement of hemodynamics [8]. In another study the vasodilator molsidomine was used first with metoprolol following it [12]. The results emphasized the importance of considering the relative

Nitroglycerin 5

contribution of the three types of myocardium, mentioned above, to global function. Ischemic myocardium improves markedly with betablockade and in a synergistic way with venous vasodilators. If only relatively small areas of functioning, non-ischemic myocardium are still present due to large scars vasodilators are necessary to counteract the impairment of contractility rendered by betablockers on these areas. If there is definite ischemia during exercise, the positive action of betablocker may become more prominent, but still is markedly enhanced by venous vasodilators.

For certain groups of patients, e.g. with hypertension after myocardial infarction, where betablockers should be used for the treatment of blood pressure as well as for "myocardial protection" a fixed combination of this drug with a nitrate may be useful. A possible negative inotropic effect of the betablocker would be balanced by the reduction of preload by the venous vasodilator. The latter would do no harm, but be advantageous for patients with reduced ventricular function, of which exact data are frequently not available. The principal advantage of the combination of a betablocker with a preload-reducing agent was shown earlier for betablockade and furosemide [6].

In the first study, presented here, a fixed combination of 40 mg ISDN in retarded form and 150 mg bupranolol was evaluated for its acute effect on ventricular function with RNV. A longer treatment period of 3 weeks followed and was controlled by exercise ECG and echocardiography.

Calcium entry blockers are also used like betablockers for both indications, hypertension and angina pectoris. They also claim "myocardial protection". Since the antianginal property often is less prominent than that of venous vasodilators and perhaps betablockers, combinations of calcium entry blockers with the other types of drugs seem warranted. Also, the occasional steal effect of arterial vasodilators like nifedipine may possibly be mitigated.

Therefore in another study we examined the effect of nifedipine before and after the addition of Molsidomine. Molsidomine, besides its similar pharmacologic profile to nitrates, seems to have less problems with tolerance development and thus does not require special time tables of application [3]. Both drugs act mainly on the vascular system, less, if at all on the myocardium. After our previous, favorable experience with a combination of molsidomine and metoprolol [14, 16] and in the light of the increasing frequency of use of combinations, it seemed worth while, to examine the relative contribution of a venous and an arterial dilatator on ventricular function. The question was to be answered, if 4 mg molsidomine still change ventricular function after administration of 10 mg nifedipine and in what way patients with and without ischemia differ in the parameters studied.

Methods

Patient selection

In the bupranolol/ISDN study, 22 consecutive outpatients, mean age 54 years, with proven coronary artery disease were studied. Within this group of 22 patients, the diagnosis of myocardial infarction was established in 11 pts. Also eleven patients showed ST-depression of 0.1 mV flat or downsloping and 11 patients had hypertension. Mean exercise level was 88 W.

In the nifedipine/molsidomine study, 19 patients, mean age 60 years, were examined. 9 patients displayed signs of ischemia on the exercise ECG with typical angina. Mean ST-depression 0.23 mV. Mean exercise level of all patients was 93 W.

Radionuclideventriculography

For the assessment of left ventricular function, RNV was performed as described elsewhere [1, 2, 4, 5, 17]. Briefly, the following procedure was employed: As a tracer erythrocytes of the pts were labeled with 20 mCi of 99 m Technetium. After intravenous administration and homogeneous distribution of the tracer, a gamma camera (Siemens LEM with computer system DEC MDA 11) was positioned in a modified 30° left anterior oblique (LAO) position. We used a matrix of 64×64 image points. Cyclic precordial variations of radioactivity correspond to cyclic volume changes of the heart chambers. Time-activity curves were recorded for each image point of the matrix, and an average curve for the left ventricle. Time resolution in this study was 32 images/heart cycle. The time-activity curve describes changes in count rate originating from the ventricles during the cardiac cycle, and reflects changes in ventricular volume between systole and diastole.

Ejection fraction was computed by dividing the difference between count rates at enddiastole and endsystole by the count rate at end-diastole after subtraction of the background.

Regional wall motion was determined by analyzing amplitudes and phases of the base frequency of the available regional time-activity curves. The diastolic borders of the right and left ventricles as well as of the atria and great vessels are delineated automatically. The magnitude of amplitude is colorcoded. The resulting normal pattern of amplitude distribution is compromised in patients with regional wall motion abnormalities. This could be shown with analysis obtained from left ventricular contrast angiography [11].

Following acquisition of the resting RNV the patients performed supine leg exercise on a bicycle ergometer. All drugs were stopped 36 hours before the first stress test. Exercise was carried out at a constant, individualized work load previously determined to consistently evoke signs of ischemia within 2–3 minutes in patients with angina pectoris or dyspnea or exhaustion after 6–8 minutes. The patients exercised about 3 minutes before the camera was started. Data collection lasted about 3–5 minutes. Systemic blood pressure was measured by a sphygmomanometer at rest and at 2 minute intervals during exercise. The precordial ECG leads V1, V5 and V6 were recorded simultaneously. Angina pectoris was graded in 3 steps, light, increasing and severe angina, enforcing to stop the exercise.

Protocol ISDN/bupranolol study

In the first group of patients TM-echocardiography was performed before exercise without medication. It was technically possible in 14 patients. Routine, supine, stepwise (25 W/step) exercise ECG was done on the bicycle ergometer to determine the symptomlimited exercise level. The first dose of the ISDN/bupranolol combination was given after the RNV control examinations at rest and during exercise. RNV was repeated after 2 hours in same manner. The patients received 2 times daily this combination of 40 mg retarded ISDN and 150 mg bupranolol. After 7 days a clinical and ECG examination was done and at the 21st day of medication echocardiography, RNV at rest and during exercise was repeated.

Protocol nifedipine/molsidomine study

In these 19 patients control RNV was performed at rest and during exercise at constant work load at a level determined like in the other group. After the control study 10 mg nifedipine were administered sublingually. Twenty minutes later the resting RNV was started with the exercise study following it at 30 min after medication with the same work load as before. After the end of exercise 4 mg Molsidomine were administered sublingually. After twenty minutes resting and exercise RNV were repeated in the same manner as before.

Statistics

Data are given as mean values with standard deviation. Statistical significance of the data was calculated using the Friedmann test for the three samples and the Wilcoxon-

Wilcox test. For comparison of the two drugs of the second study the U-Test was used. A p-value of less than 0.05 was regarded as statistically significant.

Results

In the **bupranolol/ISDN** study heart rate and blood pressure declined particularly during exercise. ST-segment depression also were reduced significantly (fig. 1). Mean exercise tolerance increased from 88 W to 105 W.

Ventricular function showed slight improvement at rest in an increase of EF from 64.5% to 66.5% (n.s.). During exercise improvement of EF from 62.9% to 66.1% was significant (p 0.01) (fig. 2, tab. 1). Enddiastolic volume decreased not significantly by 3.2% at rest and 5.1% during exercise.

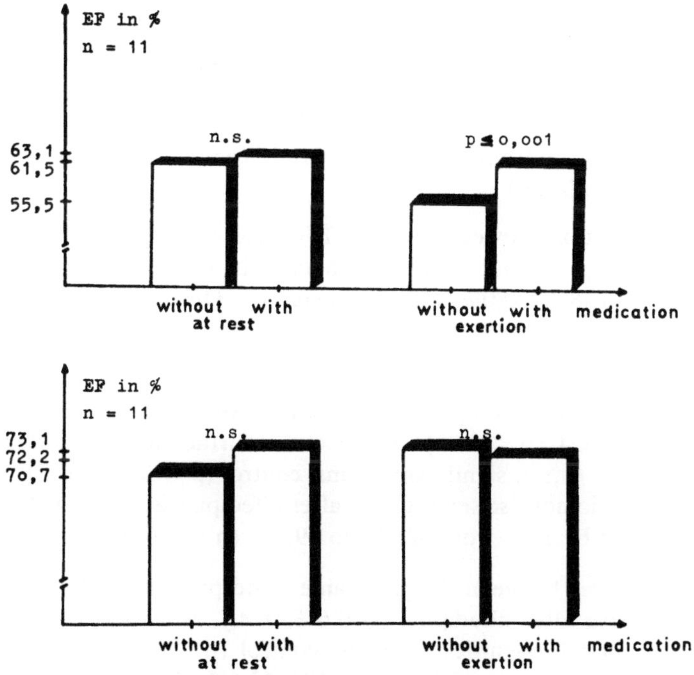

Fig. 1 Global ejection fraction (EF) at rest and during exercise before and after Bupranolol and ISDN of patients with ischemic signs in the upper part and without ischemic signs in the inferior part. An improvement of the ejection fraction could be demonstrated only in the presence of ischemia.

Echocardiographic parameters showed in 14 patients a decrease of endsystolic and enddiastolic diameters, resulting in an increase of shortening fraction by 15.6% (p 0.05).

Plasma levels of ISDN and its metabolites showed high levels over 5 hours without a clear decline of the plasma level curve of IS-5-MN during this time. ISDN showed a maximum after 2 hours, the metabolites at about 4 hours.

The results show the widening of the therapeutic range of the combination of ISDN and bupranolol. In spite of a relatively high dose of the betablocker there was no decrease of EF at rest and neither during exercise after the drugs. Also after 21 days of treatment no deterioration of left ventricular function or clinical efficacy could be detected.

Two patients had to be excluded from the study due to complaints typical for hypotension. Blood pressure was in the lower normal range. One patient had to stop medication due to bradycardia.

In the **nifedipine/molsidomine** study heart rate rose at rest from 65/min to 75/min after nifedipine and to 81/min after molsidomine significantly. Since the time between exercises is relatively short, comparison of resting values is not quite representative for a heart rate effect of the drugs. During exercise mean heart rate increased only after nifedipine from 104/min to 111/min (p 0.05), after molsidomine it remained unchanged (112/min).

Results from ejection fraction showed a range of EF at rest from 26% to 82%, mean value 66.8% in the group without exercise ischemia. In the group with signs of ischemia EF ranged from 48% to 80%, mean value 62.4%. During exercise mean EF hardly changed in the group without ischemia to 65.3%, whereas in the other group with ischemia it decreased to 52.1%.

In the group without ischemia nifedipine showed a relative increase of EF of 6.3% from 66.8% to 71% at rest ($p < 0.05$). There was a further increase after molsidomine at rest to 74.4% (n.s.), significant against control ($p < 0.01$, fig. 2). In the group with ischemia EF did not rise significantly after nifedipine at rest (fig. 3). After molsidomine it increased by 11% from 62.3% to 69.2% ($p < 0.01$).

During exercise differences between drugs became more prominent. In the group without ischemia EF rose after nifedipine by 6.6% (n.s.). After molsidomine EF increased by 15% to 74.4%, significant against control ($p < 0.01$, fig. 3). In the group with ischemia during exercise EF increased by 12.6% after nifedipine (n.s.), after molsidomine a further increase by 17.4% from 58.7% to 68.9% was observed. This was significant against control ($p < 0.01$), but also against nifedipine ($p < 0.05$, fig. 3).

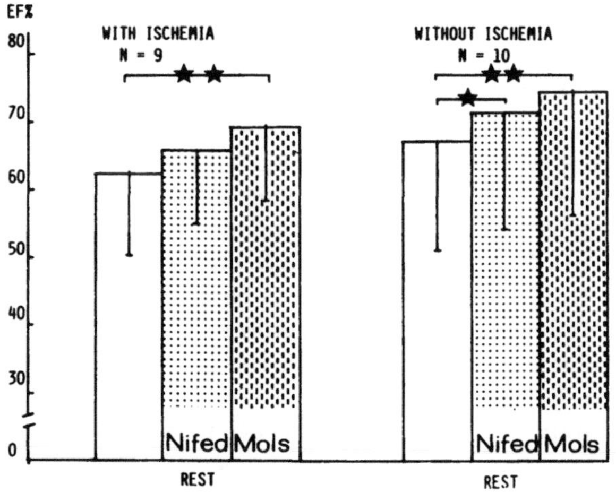

Fig. 2 Global ejection fraction of 9 patients with exercise ischemia and 10 patients without ischemia at control, after 10 mg Nifedipine s.l. and additionally after 4 mg Molsidomine s.l.

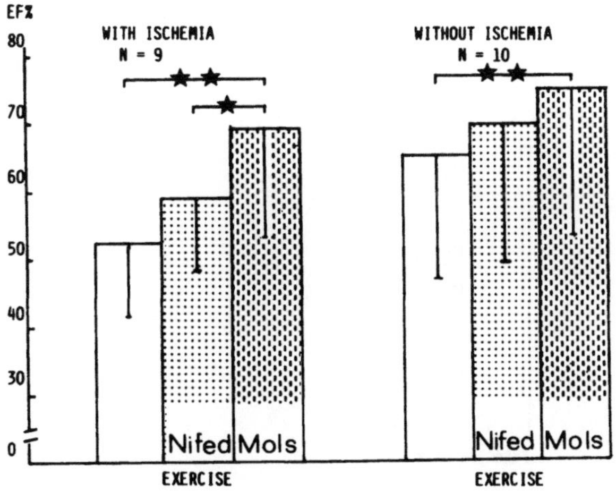

Fig. 3 Same patients as in figure 2, but during exercise.

Comparing values of EF of all 19 patients after nifedipine against values after nifedipine plus molsidomine a highly significant increase is evident, moderate in extent at rest, more marked during exercise ($p < 0.001$, fig. 4).

This result of further improvement of EF by molsidomine after nifedipine may be interpreted as a consequence of different mechanisms of action. The preload reducing action of molsidomine is still effecting an increase of EF notwithstanding the – probably mostly afterload reducing – action of nifedipine. Taking both drug effects together the increase of EF in the group with ischemia amounts to 32.4%, in the group without ischemia 14.1%. It does not seem to be an effect of inadequate dosing. In an earlier study we administered 20 mg nifedipine s.l. in an interindividual comparison with 4 mg molsidomine [15]. The range of change of EF was similar to this study with 10 mg nifedipine: Increase of EF at rest by 8.1% and during exercise by 10% (relative %). Contrary to this study, however, there was a significant increase of heart rate during exercise after 20 mg nifedipine. Taking into account a possible difference in patient's disease state and a different effect on heart rate, there seems to be no conclusive evidence that 20 mg of nifedipine would change EF any more than 10 mg.

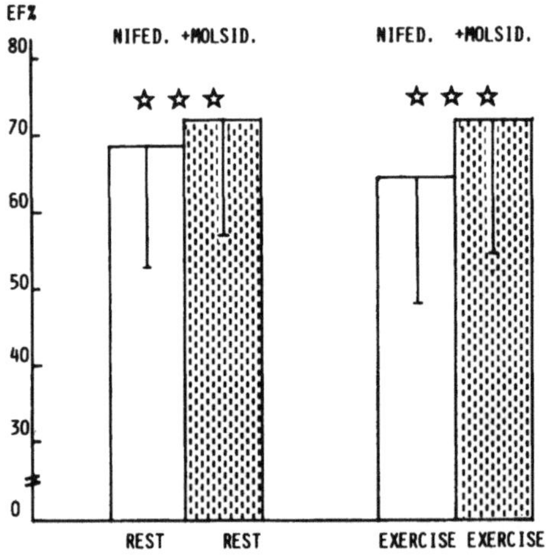

Fig. 4 Comparison of the ejection fraction of all 19 patients (fig. 2 and 3) at rest and during exercise after Nifedipine and after Nifedipine and Molsidomine, respectively.

Conclusion

The use of combinations of venous vasodilators ISDN and molsidomine with bupranolol or nifedipine is useful and recommendable in patients with coronary heart disease. Patients with marked ischemia during exercise usually show adequate ventricular function at rest and a clear deterioration during exercise. The anti-ischemic effect, as measured by improvement of left ventricular function during exercise, is enhanced by both combination of these antianginal drugs. In patients without significant signs of ischemia during exercise but impaired ventricular function at rest without much change during exercise function is improved by nifedipine and further significantly improved by the addition of the vasodilator molsidomine. The use of ISDN and bupranolol in a fixed combination on these patients without ischemia leaves EF unchanged, a decrease of EF by the betablocker alone would be expected.

References

[1] Adam, W. E., A. Tarkowsky, F. Bitter et al.: Equilibrium (gated) radionuclide ventriculography. Cardiovasc. Radiol. **2** (1979) 161.

[2] Borer, J. S., S. L. Bacharach, M. V. Green et al.: Real-time radionuclide cineangiography in the n-oninvasive evaluation of global and regional left ventricular function at rest and during exercise in patients with coronary artery disease. N. Engl. J. Med. **296** (1977) 839–844.

[3] Brügmann, U., R. Blasini, W. Rudolph: Die Wirkung von Molsidomin auf den Pulmonalarteriendruck bei Patienten mit chronischer Herzinsuffizienz und auf die ST-Streckensenkung bei Patienten mit Angina pectoris. Med. Klin. Suppl. **1** (1985) 54–57.

[4] Geffers, H., H. Sigel, F. Bitter et al.: Untersuchungen der segmentalen Wandbewegung des linken Ventrikels bei Herzgesunden und Myokardinfarktpatienten mit einer katheterlosen nuklearmedizinischen Methode (Kamera-Kinematographie des Herzens). Z. Kardiol. **65** (1976) 680–692.

[5] Geffers, H., W. E. Adam, F. Bitter et al.: Radionuklid-Ventrikulographie I. Grundlagen und Methode. Nucl.-Med. **17** (1978) 206–210.

[6] Nechwatal, W., H. Sigel, F. Bitter et al.: Die globale und regionale Funktion des linken Ventrikels bei koronarer Herzerkrankung nach Betablockade und Furosemid. Dtsch. Wochenschr. **105** (1980) 1687–1693.

[7] Nechwatal, W., M. Stauch, H. Sigel et al.: Effects of Molsidomine on global and regional left ventricular function at rest and during exercise in patients with angina pectoris. Clin. Cardiol. **4** (1981) 248–253.

[8] Nechwatal, W.: Die Ventrikelfunktion bei Patienten mit Angina pectoris. Einfluß von β-adrenerger Blockade und Nitraten. Springer, Berlin–Heidelberg–New York–Tokio 1984.

[9] Pfisterer, M., J. Müller-Brand, F. Burkart et al.: Combined acebutolol/nifedipine therapy in patients with chronic coronary artery disease: additional improvement of ischemia-induced left ventricular dysfunction. Am. J. Cardiol. **49** (1982) 1259.

[10] Richter, P., H. Sigel, W. Nechwatal et al.: Vergleich der enddiastolischen Volumina des linken Ventrikels bestimmt mittels der Radionuklidventrikulographie, der Kontrastmittelventrikulographie und einer geometrieunabhängigen Methode. Z. Kardiol. **75** (1986).

[11] Sigel, H., H. Geffers, P. Kress et al.: Über die Erfassung regionaler Funktionsstörungen des linken Ventrikels durch nuklearmedizinische Methoden. Herz/Kreisl. **11** (1979) 102.

[12] Stauch, M., P. Kress, W. E. Adam: Assessment of the effect of ISDN and its metabolites on ventricular function at rest and during exercise by radionuclideventriculography, Brit. J. Clin. Pract. Suppl. **26** (1983) 59–67.

[13] Stauch M., P. Kress, H. Geffers et al.: Influence of isosorbide dinitrate and mononitrate on the ejection fraction and wall motion paramaters at rest and under exercise in patients with coronary heart disease. In: Nitrates III (P. R. Lichtlen et al., eds.). Springer, Berlin–Heidelberg–New York 1981.

[14] Stauch, M., W. Haerer, G. Rogg-Dussler et al.: Effects of molsidomine on reginal contraction and global function of the left ventricle. Am. Heart. J. **109** (1985a) 653–658.

[15] Stauch, M. T. Hermann, J. Roth et al.: Die Wirkung von Molsidomin und Nifedipin auf die Funktion des linken Ventrikels bei Patienten mit koronarer Herzkrankheit. Med. Klinik Suppl. **1** (1985b) 34–38.

[16] Stauch, M., W. Nechwatal, P. Kress, H. Sigel, F. Bitter, W. E. Adam: Die Wirkung von Molsidomin und Metoprolol auf die Auswurffraktion des linken Ventrikels in Ruhe und während Belastung bei Patienten mit koronarer Herzkrankheit. In: Molsidomin, Neue Aspekte zur Therapie der ischämischen Herzerkrankung (E. Bassenge, H. Schmutzler, eds.). Urban & Schwarzenberg, München–Wien–Baltimore 1982.

[17] Stauch, M., H. Sigel, H. Geffers et al.: Radionuklidventrikulographie. II Klinische Ergebnisse: Parameter der globalen Ventrikelfunktion. Nucl. Med. **17** (1978) 211.

Nitrate tolerance

H. Just

Introduction

Soon after nitrates were first introduced as a form of treatment some 140 years ago it was noticed that their effect decreased on repeated administration. In 1888 Stewart described the phenomenon of nitrate tolerance with great clarity. To maintain the initial reduction in his blood pressure, one of Stewart's patients finally required two thousand times the original dose. The reversible nature of tolerance was also discovered at an early stage; it was found that workers in explosives factories, who had become tolerant during the week through inhalation at their jobs, reacted when they started work again after the weekend, sometimes with severe symptoms.

There is no doubt today that tolerance to nitrates can be induced in a reproducible form experimentally and in a clinical setting through suitable application and dosage. Whether the development of tolerance is significant in the clinical situation is, however, a matter of controversy.

The aim of this paper is to consider the mechanisms of tolerance development and then to demonstrate their clinical importance.

Mechanisms of tolerance development

A reduction or complete loss of therapeutic efficacy, that is of nitrate-induced vasodilatation, can come about in various ways.

1. Pseudotolerance through counterregulation: The predominantly venous dilatation induced by nitrates leads to a reduction of cardiac stroke volume and thus to a fall in blood pressure even at dosages at which arteriolar dilatation does not yet occur. The sympathetic counterregulation via the baroreceptors which then begins increases the heart rate and the contractile performance of the myocardium. At very low doses a reactive vasoconstriction in the arterioles can also be observed. This quickly compensates for an initial fall in blood pressure and attenuates the potency of the nitrates as vasodilators at the arteriolar level.

Nitroglycerin 5

In cases of congestive heart failure with a high filling potential of the left ventricle there is no reduction of stroke volume due to preload reduction. The baroreceptor reflex is not activated. Counterregulation occurs directly at the ventricular level. The effect of nitrates is present in such cases. Blood pressure and heart rate are not suitable parameters for measurement.

2. The vasodilator capacity of nitrates may cease when there is increased extravascular resistance. In hydropic heart failure the nitrates may fail to act from the beginning or cease to act if there is increased retention of fluid during nitrate treatment. Such an effect may even be observed under high-dose nitrate treatment (acting on the arterioles) when the renin-angiostens in-aldosterone system is activated and an increased amount of fluid is retained.

A loss of effect due to haemodynamic factors may also occur when increased amounts of extracellular fluid enter the venous system during predominantly venous dilatation (low nitrate doses), thus enlarging the intravenous blood volume. It is probable that via this mechanism the vasodilator capacity of the nitrates can first be interrupted in the abdominal area, thus causing a fall-off in effect.

3. Development of tolerance in the true sense of the term: The effect of nitrates at cellular level consists in the fact that when the substance has entered the cell it is broken down into nitrosothiols under the influence of glutathione reductase. The nitrosothiols directly activate the formation of guanylate cyclase which is of decisive importance for vasodilatation, for it converts GTP into cyclic GMP; it is this that directly induces relaxation of the smooth vascular muscle.

An increased breakdown rate of the nitrates brought about by glutathione reductase by way of enzymatic reduction has been discussed as an important mechanism of tolerance development: it was said that induction of this enzyme in the liver led to increased breakdown in the first pass effect and thus to a loss of effectiveness after peroral application. Today it may be regarded as established that an increasing first pass effect is of no consequence in the development of tolerance. On the other hand tolerance may well be explained by biochemical processes in the vascular muscle cells. The formation of nitrosothiols by glutathione reductase requires the presence of glutamyl-cysteinylglycine. As long as the latter is not fully oxidised to glutathione disulphide it enables the reduction of the nitrates and thus vasodilatation through an increase in guanylate cyclase and CGMP. But as soon as the stock is exhausted no further nitrate is reduced and vascular dilatation ceases. Elegant in vitro investigations have shown that this loss of effect can be counteracted by the introduction of cysteine. In patients, too, it proved possible to considerably intensify the effect of nitroglycerin by administering N-acetylcysteine. This mechanism, which is probably of fundamental importance in the development of tolerance, is dose-related and can be influenced or regenerated (administration of sulphide-groups?).

Finally, a further proof that these mechanisms are indeed responsible for the development of tolerance may be seen in the fact that there are substances (molsidomine, Sin 1 A) capable of increasing the guanylate cyclase and thus the cyclic GMP by acting "behind" the nitrosothiol stage. These do not develop tolerance.

Partial tolerance

It has long been known that the typical nitrate headache can disappear without a loss of anti-anginal efficacy. We must therefore ask ourselves whether the effect of nitrates may differ in the various vascular provinces.

It is known that venous dilatation can be achieved with much lower nitrate doses than arteriolar dilatation. What we do not know for certain is whether regional, organ-related vascular provinces react in different ways. The greatest attention has so far been devoted to the coronary system, but first studies of the splanchnic system are now being submitted. Comparisons of effect on the coronary, cerebral and renal or other organ-related vascular regions are not yet available or the findings are not yet sufficiently verified. It may however be that the venous pooling effect caused by the inflow of extra-vascular fluid is most likely to cease in the splanchnic region.

Development of tolerance and the nitrate plasma level

The higher the nitrate plasma level, the earlier and the more pronounced is the onset of tolerance. At values above 500 ng/ml tolerance is to be expected regularly. At levels below 100, and even more so below 50 ng/ml, tolerance development is rare or slight.

The clinical studies carried out by Rudolf and by Parker also suggest that the development of nitrate tolerance is dependent on the plasma level. Rudolf et al. administered 40 mg of ISDN four times daily, Parker 15 mg four times daily. In both cases tolerance to the acute administration of 5 mg ISDN sublingually developed within a maximum of 48 hours. After the peroral ISDN had been discontinued or replaced by a placebo the acute effect of sublingual ISDN was restored within 20 hours. These observations are compatible with the assumption that the development of tolerance is related to the plasma level. Parker therefore recommended giving the nitrate for only six to ten hours per day in therapeutically effective doses and allowing a period of 14 to 18 hours with low plasma levels before the next tablets were taken. Silver tested this recommendation and found that 80 mg ISDN given once daily in slow-release form was still effective after a fortnight, whilst 80 mg twice daily in standard-release form led to a complete loss of effect.

If nitrate plasma levels are compared at different doses and at different times it is possible to establish fairly exactly the boundary between tolerance and continued effectiveness.

On the basis of the elimination constant, absorption constant, volume of distribution, bio-availability, administered dose (per tablet), number of tablets per day and the length of treatment in days, it is possible to calculate blood level courses in advance and then to elaborate dosage recommendations for the various nitrate preparations that promise good clinical efficacy and prevent the development of tolerance as far as possible.

Clinical significance

The nitrates are used mainly to treat coronary heart disease with angina pectoris and for the treatment of heart failure. In both cases the nitrates are both used to control acute manifestations (angina, acute left heart failure) as well as for long-term therapy.

Coronary heart disease: It is typical of myocardial ischaemia that it occurs intermittently. Intermittent application of nitrates before, at the onset of, during or immediately after an attack is effective and not impaired by tolerance. Long-term application is only advisable if the ischaemic attacks are frequent or if the underlying disease can be influenced by the establishment of a permanently elevated nitrate plasma level. There is, however, no proof of this so far. On the contrary, a permanent effect is only desirable in the case of beta blockers (prevention of sudden myocardial infarction or reinfarction) and calcium antagonists (myocardial protection, vascular protection). Only if angina attacks are very frequent, or in a state of unstable angina, is a long-term effect (more than 24 hours) of therapeutic importance.

The reason why the phenomenon of tolerance has not been so apparent in the past is probably that the mode of application was intermittent even for long-term treatment (short-lasting effect of the preparation) and that the ischaemic condition only occurs intermittently. Not until the development of modes of application inducing a permanently high blood level (infusion, transdermal plaster preparations) did the question of tolerance become important.

As tolerance is provoked by all nitrate preparations but can, on the other hand, be diminished by application at intervals or by administration of slow-release forms with secondary release of effective metabolites, nitrate tolerance is a remarkable problem but one that is clinically relevant in only a few situations in coronary heart disease.

This applies in particular to unstable angina pectoris. Here a lasting coronary effect must be achieved. The recommended procedure in such cases is intermittent i.v. administration, elimination of factors promoting the development of tolerance (see above), or use of nitrate-like substances that increase the guanylate cyclase concentration directly (molsidomine, Sin 1 A) circumventing the nitrosothiol stage.

Longer-term treatment with nitrates, lasting several days, might also be of clinical significance for acute myocardial infarction. There are indications that it is possible to achieve a protective effect on the myocardium under long-term nitrate treatment. If this is so, the above recommendations would apply for the use of nitrates in such a situation.

Heart Failure: According to the studies available so far the use of nitrates is restricted to acute heart failure. They should not be administered for longer than 24 hours. The best procedure is to make a break after twelve hours and then start the infusion again. In this situation it is especially important to eliminate mechanical factors that hamper the effect of the nitrates (diuresis).

So far there is no definite proof of the effectiveness of nitrates in chronic heart failure.

Summary

Nitrate tolerance is demonstrable in vitro, in animal experiments and in human beings regularly and for all nitrate preparations. There are various mechanisms for the development of tolerance. Some of them can be corrected (increase in intracellular fluid, pronounced oedemas). Others are less easily influenced (development of tolerance at intracellular level).

As tolerance plainly develops after the effect of glutathione reductase, at the stage of nitrosothiol formation, it is conceivable that at some future date substances will be developed that bring about the increase in guanylate cyclase typical of the nitrates without the above stage, thus preventing development of tolerance at this level.

In the clinical setting of coronary heart disease with intermittent ischaemic conditions (angina pectoris) and in heart failure, development of nitrate tolerance is only significant in solated cases.

Only in unstable angina, status anginosus, acute myocardial infarction and severe heart failure refractory to treatment is a long-term effect desirable and tolerance can often be prevented or evaded if the pathogenic mechanisms of tolerance development are understood.

In principle nitrates are excellently suited for intermittent administration. The size of doses and the intervals between them (influenced by the galenism of the preparation used) should take account of the mechanisms of tolerance development currently known.

New results in the field of nitrate tolerance under nitroglycerin, ISDN and ISMN

M. Tauchert, W. Jansen

Introduction

Tolerance to the effects of a drug exists when ever-shorter intervals between administrations or steadily increasing doses of the drug are required to maintain the desired therapeutic effect. In pharmacological experiments a distinction is made between the acute form of tolerance development, i.e. tachyphylaxia, and a chronic form. In clinical studies it is extremely difficult to record the development of tolerance in exact chronological terms and thus to distinguish between tachyphylaxia and a slower development of tolerance. Nor is such a distinction usually of any significance from the therapeutic point of view.

Tolerance development results from modifications in pharmacokinetics (absorption, metabolism and elimination of the drug) and in pharmacodynamics (changes to the receptors, inhibition processes). An existing tolerance to one drug may also constitute tolerance to another preparation that has not yet been applied if the second drug acts through the same system of receptors ("cross tolerance").

Even before the turn of the century, it was known that in treatment of a hypertensive crisis the high-dose administration of nitroglycerin led to a swift loss of effect, i.e. to tolerance [12]. As nitroglycerin did not achieve general acceptance as treatment for hypertensive crises in the following years and longer-acting nitrates for treating coronary heart disease were not available, the development of tolerance under nitrate influence was of no consequence in clinical practice for several decades. The problem did not become important again until nitrates were developed that remained in the plasma longer and thus acted over a longer period; these were isosorbide dinitrate in slow-release form and isorbide-5-mononitrate. Paradoxically, then, the widespread discussion of nitrate tolerance in recent years has been a result of pharmacological improvement of the nitrates.

Nitroglycerin 5

Methods of monitoring the long-term effect of drugs acting on the coronary arteries

Record of symptoms

As far as we know at present, drugs acting on the coronaries are substances whose effect is primarily symptomatic. The obvious procedure is therefore to monitor the efficacy of treatment with these substances by keeping track of the main symptom, angina pectoris. A correct assessment is only possible if the patients treated keep a reliable record of the frequency and severity of angina attacks. These records must be checked regularly by the physician in charge and used as a basis for further therapy. And this is the main disadvantage of such a method of monitoring treatment: the doctor-patient relationship with all its interactions is intensified; this obscures the boundary between pharmacological and psychological treatment. A record of consumption of nitrate capsules or spray effective in an attack must be regarded still more critically. Here the symptoms must first be noted and classified with sufficient exactness; the next stage is the patient's decision whether or not it is necessary to use the nitrate to combat an attack, and this decision is by no means free of outside influences.

Exercise electrocardiogram

An exercise electrocardiogram answers the question whether a patient has coronary disease or not with an accuracy of 80% or more. But the answer is only "yes" or "no". For monitoring treatment with substances acting on the coronaries such a simple classification of answers is not an adequate method. Even if treatment is not fully successful an attempt must be made to register intermediate levels of effectiveness. This is problematic for two reasons: firstly, it is known that a number of factors may interfere with the exercise electrocardiogram (e.g. glycoside influence, potassium deficiency) and alter the ST-segment of the electrocardiogram in an unpredictable manner. Secondly, it is very doubtful whether the ischaemia analogue of ST-segment depression is a quantitative expression of the extent of ischaemia in the myocardium. Moreover, a considerable number of patients (10 to 20 percent) with coronary heart disease clearly established angiographically do not have an ST-segment depression on the exercise electrocardiogram commensurate with the objective findings, in spite of being exerted to capacity. For these patients, then, therapy monitoring by means of exercise electrocardiogram is out of the question; accordingly such studies are always conducted with selected patients and cannot be generalised as they stand.

Work capacity

Work capacity or work tolerance is the term given to the product of the exertion level in watts on the ergometer and the duration of exertion. Its decisive quantity is plainly the duration of exertion up to the point where angina pectoris equivalents occur. If the test conditions are strictly adhered to, this parameter is easily reproducible and well-suited to monitoring the antianginal effects of coronary drugs [7]. In the English-speaking countries such tests are usually limited to determining the duration of exertion up to the occurrence of angina pectoris ("time to angina"). Generally the exertion level is left unchanged. The reproducibility of this parameter seems also to be very high [7].

Haemodynamics

The strongest haemodynamic effect of most antianginal drugs is on the capacitive vascular system, and probably pulmonary circulation is adequately representative of this. Pressure in the pulmonary system can be measured repeatedly at rest and under exertion with justifiable effort by means of a flow catheter. The reproducibility of measurements under highly varying conditions is good [2, 7]. Accordingly, analyses of pulmonary haemodynamics must also be regarded as a suitable means of monitoring antianginal therapy.

Mechanisms of nitrate tolerance development

1. Continuous high-dose administration of nitrates may stimulate their metabolism; enzyme induction in the liver is known to exist. The result is a reduction in the bioavailability of the nitrates which may be termed metabolic tolerance. In the case of isosorbide dinitrate an enzyme induction has been proved; no similar mechanisms are known in relation to isosorbide-5-mononitrate.

2. The effect of the nitrates is mediated by reactive SH groups at the receptor. The availability of these SH groups can be so far reduced through the constant demands made on them by uninterrupted nitrate administration that the receptors no longer mediate nitrate action.

3. Nitrates induce a shift of the circulating blood volume into the capacitive vascular system. If this effect is maintained constantly it must be expected that the volume lost to the arterial system will be made up for by counterregulation. This would mean a weakening of the therapeutic effect of the nitrates although the capacitive vascular

system retains its elevated volume. This component of nitrate tolerance development might be termed "physical" tolerance.

All three mechanisms of tolerance development are reversible if the administration of nitrates is interrupted to give the reactive systems involved an opportunity to recover.

Development of tolerance to different nitrates

According to our present knowledge, we may assume that the partial and overall effects of the various nitrates are largely similar; there are differences only in the chronological course of the plasma levels and their effects. Studies of tolerance are available for all nitrates in general clinical use.

Nitroglycerin

Systematic studies of the question of tolerance development under continuous nitroglycerin administration are complicated by the fact that there are usually quick changes in medication in the acute phase of a myocardial infarction. These changes are superimposed on the nitroglycerin treatment and make it difficult to monitor the latter's course.

Our own studies of patients with recent myocardial infarctions, who had received a continuous infusion of 6 mg nitroglycerin per hour, showed that complete tolerance to nitroglycerin can develop within the space of 24 hours at most [11]. It is not yet known whether the reversal of this tolerance after administration of nitroglycerin has ceased corresponds to the fall in the plasma level. The conclusion to be drawn from this for therapy must be that no matter how severe the infarction, infusion treatment with nitroglycerin must start with low doses (proceeding from 1 mg per hour). The development of tolerance which, it seems, inevitably results from continuous administration of nitroglycerin can then be warded off for some considerable time by an increase in dosage. With such "programmed" administration of nitroglycerin it should be possible to carry out infusion treatment successfully for several days.

Long-acting nitrates

Blasini et al. [1] were the first to mention that if several nitrate doses are evenly distributed over the day, treatment with isosorbide dinitrate over an extended period of time leads to almost complete tolerance. Schneider et al. [10] found the opposite; an increase in dosage from 30 mg to 480 mg ISDN per day did not lead to a degree of tolerance demonstrable by monitoring ST-segment depression under exertion. But to summarize the literature available at present, it must be said that development of nitrate tolerance during frequent administration of medium and higher doses is plainly inevitable and is also of significance to therapy.

In patients with chronic heart failure, Franciosa [3] and also Leier [8] saw that average doses of ISDN did not lead to reduced effect when applied three times daily during treatment lasting several weeks. When evaluating these findings one must take into account that patients with heart failure are usually given multiple therapy and that this probably interferes with the nitrate treatment. Diuretics, in particular, are likely to be a factor here.

Our own studies have shown that daily administration of 60 mg ISDN or 60 mg IS-5-MN (in three portions) does not lead to a reduction in effect significant for therapy within a period of four weeks [5]. But the same regimen regularly results in tolerance if the dose is increased threefold. The dose-effect relationship cannot be taken as a reason for giving such high doses (see fig. 1).

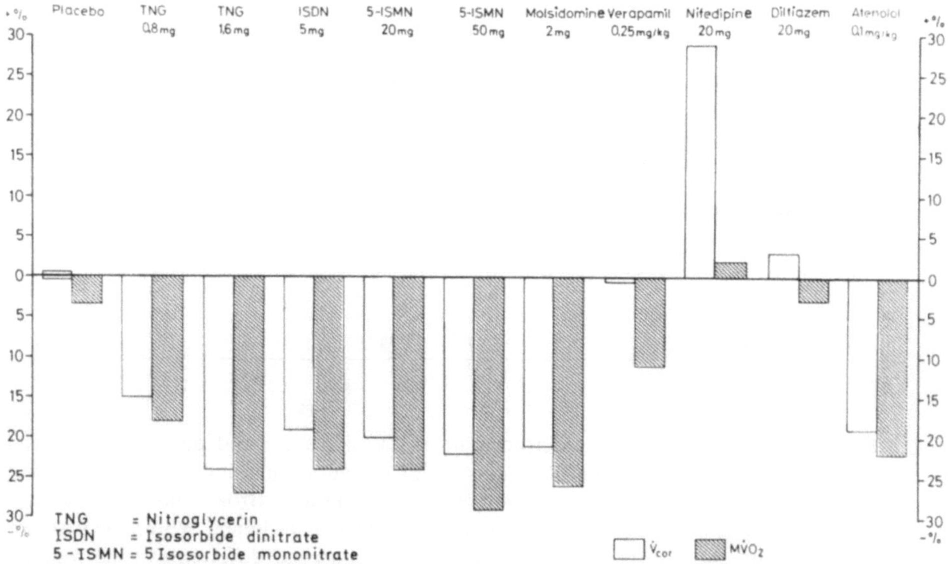

Fig. 1 Table showing the effect of various nitrates and other drugs acting on the coronaries on myocardial oxygen consumption and total blood supply to the myocardium (from [6]). It is of particular interest here that the increased dosage does not bring about an increase in effect proportionate to the dose with either TNG or 5-ISM.

According to present information, it must be assumed that almost continual administration of oral nitrates leads to a loss of effect which is probably less dependent on the size of the dose than on the absence of "intervals for recovery". Two possible solutions are to give constantly higher doses or to interrupt nitrate administration frequently. In long-term treatment the only reasonable course is to create intervals by interrupting the intake of nitrates. ISDN and IS-5-MN behave identically in this respect, as a metabolite of ISDN decisive for long-term action is also IS-5-MN. As far as we can tell from the studies available at present, losses of effect are to be expected from the eighth to twelfth hour onwards if the nitrate-plasma level remains constant. Within approximately 24 hours a continuously-maintained plasma concentration results in self-inhibition of the nitrates. In the interest of effective long-term therapy, therefore, it is necessary to bring the nitrate-plasma concentration down below the therapeutically effective level each day, probably for several hours. This does not necessarily mean that a plasma concentration of almost zero must be reached.

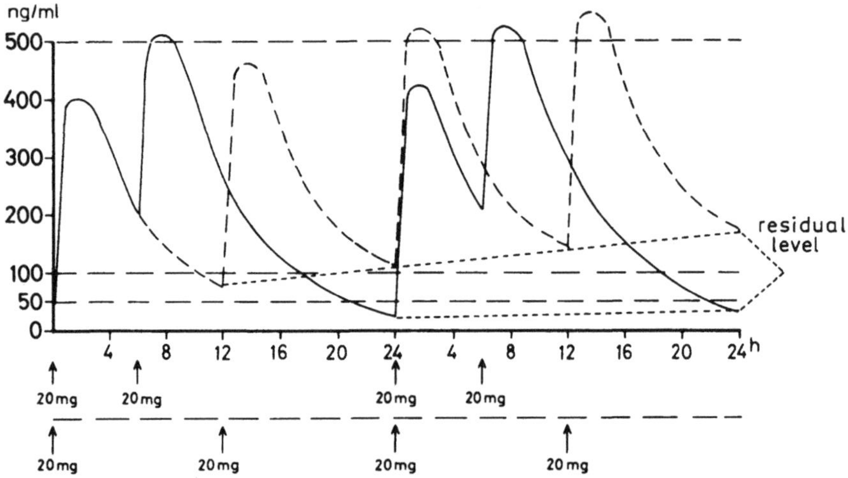

Fig. 2 Plasma level courses calculated from data in the literature and our own results on application of 2×20 mg IS-5-MN per day [14]. Continuous line: intake at time 0 and at time 0 plus 6 hours followed by an 18-hour break in intake. Broken line: plasma level course on intake of 20 mg IS-5-MN at time 0 and at 0 plus 12 hours. Within the first two days of treatment with the same total dose there is a clear difference in the residual levels resulting from different application. This difference does not continue in the same measure during a longer period of treatment and it is likely that its significance for therapy is slight. It does, however, show that nitrates with high bio-availability require precise planning and conduct of medication.

Figure 2 shows how sensitive the relationship between applied dose, intervals between doses, and plasma levels is, provided that no variations in the plasma level course result from pharmacokinetic factors.

Nitroglycerin plasters

Nitroglycerin plasters were originally regarded more or less as a placebo, as in most prescriptions they were applied in addition to an oral nitrate therapy of longer standing. Studies of plasma levels have, however, shown that if the plasters adhere well the required plasma concentrations can in fact be maintained for almost 24 hours [4]. The dose-effect relationship for the doses used here is good [13]. Parker and Fung were the first to prove [9] that under administration of nitroglycerin by means of plasters, therapeutically relevant losses of effect occur even during the first few hours. Continuous medication from plasters through application without a break maintains total tolerance. The only conclusion to be drawn from this is that contrary to general therapeutic recommendations, plasters should not be used for 24 hours with immediate renewal; if at all, they should only be used for the therapeutically important half of the day.

Conclusions for the use of nitrates

The above findings and deliberations lead us to make the following recommendations for nitrate treatment:

1. Treatment should always begin with the lowest doses that may be expected to produce an effect. In the case of nitroglycerin, this dose should be about 1 mg per hour or less; in the case of isosorbide dinitrate and IS-5-MN, 20 mg or less.

2. The individual doses should be distributed in such a way that there is a break of several hours each day in nitrate administration in accordance with the pharmacokinetic properties of the substance used. A break does not mean that the plasma level of the particular preparation or its effective metabolites reaches zero.

3. If an increase in dosage seems unavoidable in a particular case, care must be taken that intervals occur although the plasma levels to be expected are high. This means that an interval of at least 12 hours must be ensured between the last intake on the previous day and the first intake on the following day.

4. If a patient does not respond adequately to standard nitrate doses, a combination with other coronary drugs should be considered rather than an increase in the nitrate dose.

Requirements for further research

The parameters used so far to monitor a possible development of tolerance are not generally accepted. On the other hand it would lead to an unreasonable selection of a few patients if, in the case of each patient, several parameters had to change in the same direction. It should, however, be a requirement that studies on the problem of tolerance development must contain, as far as possible, two parameters independent of each other but having to react in the same direction for the results to be accepted as proof. Such a combination of test parameters would seem more sensible than rigid insistence on randomization and double blind studies.

The studies carried out so far on dose-effect relationships of nitrates or on thresholds for plasma concentrations were conducted in the phase of equilibrium of nitrate kinetics or at the peak nitrate level. Additional investigations of the falling side of the plasma-level curve, which accounts for a major part of the drug's action time, are urgently needed.

Furthermore, it is still uncertain whether origin and suppression of spontaneous angina attacks can be influenced therapeutically in the same manner as the symptoms under conditions of exertion. This question is especially topical in view of recent increased discussion on silent myocardial ischaemia. But at this point difficulties of method arise, as the methods that can be used to record spontaneous or silent ischaemia cannot be accepted without reservation. The technical standard of the monitoring systems available at present certainly does not permit us to formulate suggestions for therapy in cases of silent ischaemia. However, it is not out of the question that new, established information on the origins of spontaneous or silent myocardial ischaemia will challenge the validity of the therapeutic suggestions formulated here.

References

[1] Blasini, R., U. Brügmann, A. Mannes et al.: Wirksamkeit von Isosorbiddinitrat in retardierter Form bei Langzeitbehandlung. Herz **5** (1980) 298.

[2] Burkart, F., S. Barold, E. Sowton: Hemodynamic effect of repeated exercise. Am. J. Cardiol. **20** (1967) 509.

[3] Franciosa, J. A., J. Y. Cohn: Sustained hemodynamic effect without tolerance during longterm isosorbide dinitrate treatment of chronic left ventricular failure. Am. J. Cardiol. **45** (1980) 648.

[4] Gerardin, A., D. Gaudry, J. Moppert et al.: Glycerol trinitrate (nitroglycerin) plasma concentrations achieved after application of transdermal therapeutic systems to healthy volunteers. Arzneim.-Forschung **35** (1985) 530.

[5] Jansen, W., A. Osterspey, M. Tauchert et al.: 5-Isosorbidmononitrat unter Ruhe- und Belastungsbedingungen bei koronarer Herzkrankheit. Dtsch. Med. Wochenschr. **107** (1982) 1499.

[6] Jansen, W., M. Tauchert, A. Osterspey et al.: Systemische und koronare Haemodynamik bei Elantan® 20 und 50. In: Mononitrat III (Eds. H. Hochrein, M. Tauchert, A. Schrey, M. Weiss), p. 38. Dr. C. Wolf & Sohn, München 1984.

[7] Jansen, W., M. Behnke, A. Osterspey et al.: Reproduzierbarkeit und Placeboanfälligkeit von Belastungsuntersuchungen mittels Einschwemmkatheter. Herz/Kreislauf **10** (1985) 529.

[8] Leier, C. V., P. Huss, R. D. Magorien et al.: Improved exercise capacity and differing arterial and venous tolerance during chronic isosorbide dinitrate therapy for congestive heart failure. Circulation **67** (1983) 817.

[9] Parker, J. O., H. L. Fung: Transdermal nitroglycerin in angina pectoris. Am. J. Cardiol. **54** (1984) 471.

[10] Schneider, W., B. Stahl, M. Kaltenbach et al.: Dosis-Wirkungs-Beziehung bei der Behandlung der Angina pectoris mit Isosorbiddinitrat. Dtsch. Med. Wochenschr. **107** (1982) 771.

[11] Schulz, V., W. Jansen, E. Pöhler et al.: Toleranz gegen Nitroglyzerin bei mehrtägiger intravenöser Zufuhr. Verh. dtsch. Ges. inn. Med. **88** (1982) 669.

[12] Stewart, D. D.: Tolerance to nitroglycerine. JAMA **44** (1905) 1678.

[13] Tauchert, M., W. Jansen, A. Osterspey: Dosis-Wirkungs-Beziehung bei Anwendung von transdermalem Nitrolgyzerin aus haemodynamischer Sicht. In: Depot-Nitrat (Eds. W.-D. Bussmann, A. Schrey), p. 136. Verlag für angew. Wissenschaften, München 1984.

[14] Tauchert, M., W. Jansen, A. Osterspey: Nitrate. Nitratdosen und Toleranz. In: Mononitrat IV (Eds. U. Borchard, W. Rafflenbeul, A. Schrey), p. 45, Dr. C. Wolf & Sohn, München 1985.

Current results of nitroglycerin therapy

J. O. Parker

Parker reports his current results of nitroglycerin therapy
(Editorial summary*)

Nitroglycerin sprays prepared as dose variants with 0.2 mg, 0.4 mg and 0.8 mg as well as placebo were studied for their haemodynamic and antianginal effects. The sublingual tablet typical of Northern America was also tested. The investigation was made with patients who had an established angina pectoris which could be reproduced via ergometer exercise. The study set-up was randomized, double-blind, crossover and placebo-controlled. The parameters used were time to onset of first exertion symptoms, time to appearance of angina pectoris pain which terminated the exercise, systolic blood pressure, heart rate at rest and on exertion, time to 1 mm ST-segment depression.

There was a significant rate increase at rest compared to placebo which rose with the dose. The systolic pressure also showed a significant reaction compared to placebo but without demonstrable dose dependence. For all types of dose haemodynamic efficacy was shown on exertion compared to placebo.

When exercise tolerance was measured until the first symptoms appeared, a clear dose-related increase in tolerance was revealed compared to placebo. The exertion time to moderate angina was increased in a similar way but it was not possible to objectify the dose-effect relationship between the 0.4 and 0.8 forms. The time to 1 mm ST-segment depression is significantly greater than for placebo without any demonstrable significant dose relationship for the higher dosages.

The tablet which was also tested showed comparable results on the whole to nitroglycerin spray at the 0.4 and 0.8 dosages. If the Nitrolingual® Spray were introduced to the American market, its advantage would be its many years of reliability. It was customary to throw away the open package with a few tablets still in it due to the rapid loss of active substance. This touched upon the aspect of costs. Controlling the costs was very topical also in the USA.

* (Study meanwhile publ. in: Am. J. Cardiol. **57** (1986) 1–5.)

Nitroglycerin 5

Presentation of the Nitrolingual prize, 1985

A. Boskamp

Professor Strauer,
Ladies and Gentlemen,

First of all I should like to thank Professor Strauer most sincerely for taking on the job of coordinating today's events and – as I can already see – ensuring their success. Then I wish to express my gratitude to all the speakers, some of whom have travelled long distances to be here with us. Finally I would like to take this opportunity of extending my personal thanks to my co-workers who have put in long hours of effort preparing the Symposium. Above all Mrs. Marwitz who was among those who received you outside; then Dr. Spitaler, and most particularly Mr. Rüdiger Pohlmann who has done most of the work of organization.

This Symposium coincides with the 150th anniversary of our firm. We held the actual celebrations back in the spring, but we have hung up the old and new symbols of the company as a reminder. The business has been in our family for nearly 90 years and I hope that we shall continue our work well into the future.

It gives me special pleasure to welcome numerous guests from abroad, for the congresses have so far been more or less confined to the Federal Republic of Germany. But now we have the pleasure of welcoming guests, scientists and business associates from Sweden, England, Canada, Belgium, Holland, France, Switzerland, Austria, Ireland and the USA. I cannot greet each of you individually, but I do welcome you all most warmly. I am happy to see you here.

But the main purpose of this address is, of course, to present the Nitrolingual Prize to Dr. Staritz. He is the speaker you have just heard. The committee was made up of three professors, all of whom are cardiologists: Professor Bleifeld in Hamburg, Professor Hochrein in Berlin and Professor Senges in Heidelberg. These three cardiologists have been generous enough to award the prize to a gastroenterological study, thus showing that nitrolgycerin has fields of application outside the sphere of cardiology and also that experts in cardiology acknowledge this fact.

Dr. Staritz, your impressive lecture confirms the rightness of the committee's decision. I congratulate you most cordially; here is the certificate. May I read out the title of the study again; it is in English:

Nitroglycerin 5

"The Effect of Glyceryl Trinitrate on the Intravascular Oesophageal Variceal Pressure (IOVP) Assessed under Basal Conditions and Intraabdominal Pressure Elevation".

I now present **Dr. Staritz** with the Nitrolingual Prize for 1985. We thank Dr. Staritz for his work and congratulate him on his achievement.

Supplement

Nitroglycerin prevents exercise induced regional myocardial dysfunction in dogs

W. Schneider, G. Krumpl, N. Mayer, G. Raberger

Introduction

The aim of the study was to investigate the efficacy of nitroglycerin (Nitro POHL® infus) on exercise induced regional myocardial dysfunction. Previous studies carried out in our laboratories with anesthetized dogs [1] did not show a nitroglycerin induced improvement. Therefore the antianginal efficiency of the drug was investigated in an experimental set-up mimicking the clinical situation of angina pectoris in conscious dogs [2]. Up to now, results in a similar model have been presented only using isosorbid-dinitrate.

Instrumentation

6 mongrel dogs of either sex weighing between 17 and 29 kg were trained to run on a treadmill. Chronical instrumentation was performed under aseptic conditions using pentobarbital anesthesia. For recording of left ventricular pressure and dp/dt a microtip manometer was inserted into the left ventricle via the apex. Regional myocardial function was assessed by sonomicrometry. For this, two pairs of piezoelectric ultrasonic crystals were implanted subendocardially, one in the area supplied by the left circumflex coronary artery (LCX), the other in the area supplied by the left anterior descending artery (LAD). A hydraulic occluder was placed around the LCX. Measurement of arterial blood pressure was carried out by means of a catheter advanced into the descending aorta via the left carotid artery. A catheter inserted into the right atrium from the left jugular vein served for drug infusions. All catheters and wires were exteriorized between the scapulae. The dogs recovered completely within a couple of days, but the investigations were commenced only one week after surgery (figs. 1–9).

Nitroglycerin 5

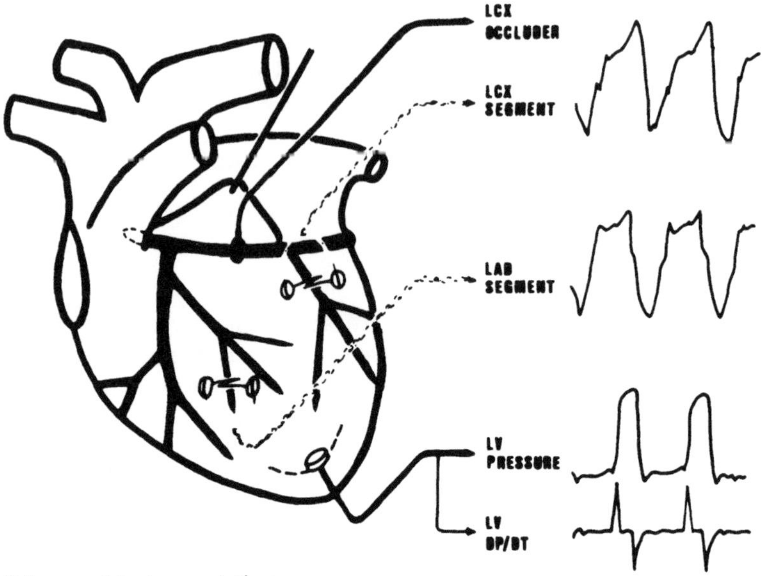

Fig. 1 Scheme of instrumentation.

Fig. 2 Treadmill exercise (LCX-stenosis) mean ± SEM, (n = 10). Hemodynamic and functional parameters at rest and during exercise.

L-LCX = segment length of the LCX area; upper curve = enddiastolic length; lower curve = endsystolic length; the height of the hatched area is equivalent to systolic shortening of the segment (SST-LCX). L-LAD = segment length in the LAD area analogous to L-LCX. TE = treadmill exercise.

Reproducibility of the exercise induced dysfunction at a constant degree of transient LCX stenosis is shown by regional contactile dysfunction of comparable magnitude in the LCX area during the 1st and 5th run after narrowing of the LCX.

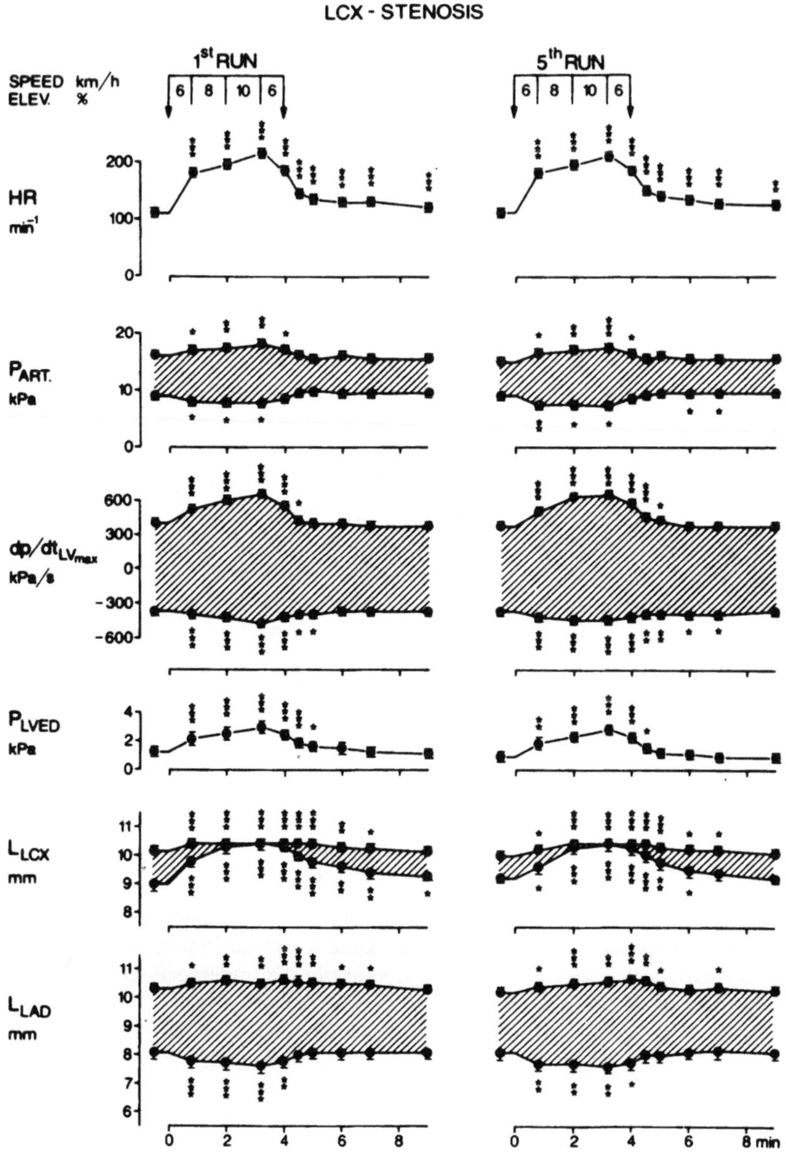
LCX - STENOSIS
1st RUN
5th RUN
SPEED km/h
ELEV. %
6 8 10 6
HR
min⁻¹
200
100
0
P ART.
kPa
20
10
dp/dt LVmax
kPa/s
600
300
-300
-600
P LVED
kPa
4
2
L LCX
mm
11
10
9
8
L LAD
mm
7
6
0
2
4
6
8
8 min

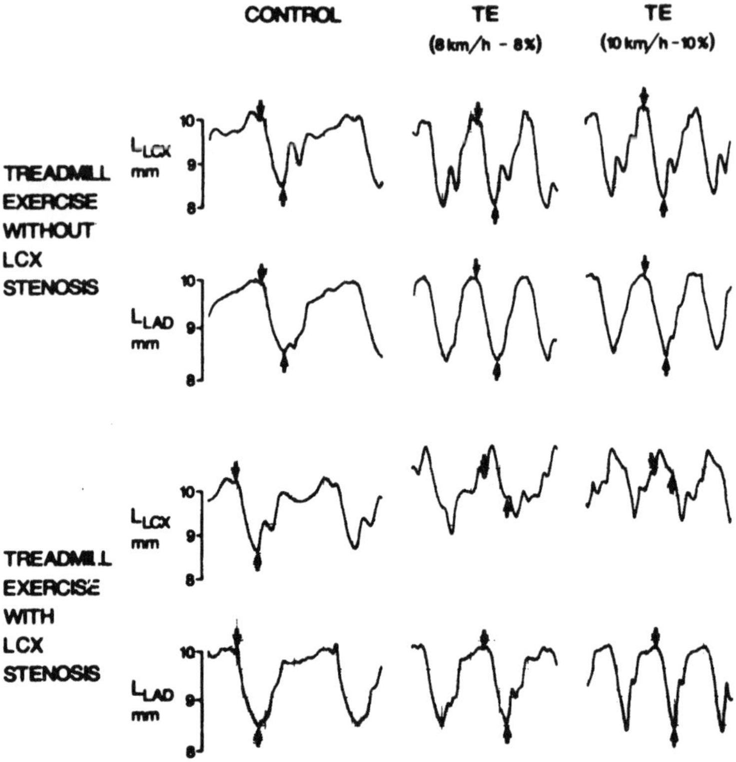

Fig. 3 Original recordings of regional myocardial shortening in the LCX- (L-LCX) and LAD area (L-LAD). Upper panel: treadmill exercise without LCX-stenosis: lower panel: treadmill exercise with LCX stenosis. ↓ : beginning of systolic shortening (= enddiastolic length); ↑ : end of systolic shortening (= endsystolic length).

In the normally perfused area (no LCX stenosis) an increased workload enhances systolic shortening. After LCX stenosis the same workload induces a regional myocardial dysfunction (decrease in systolic shortening) in the underperfused LCX area.

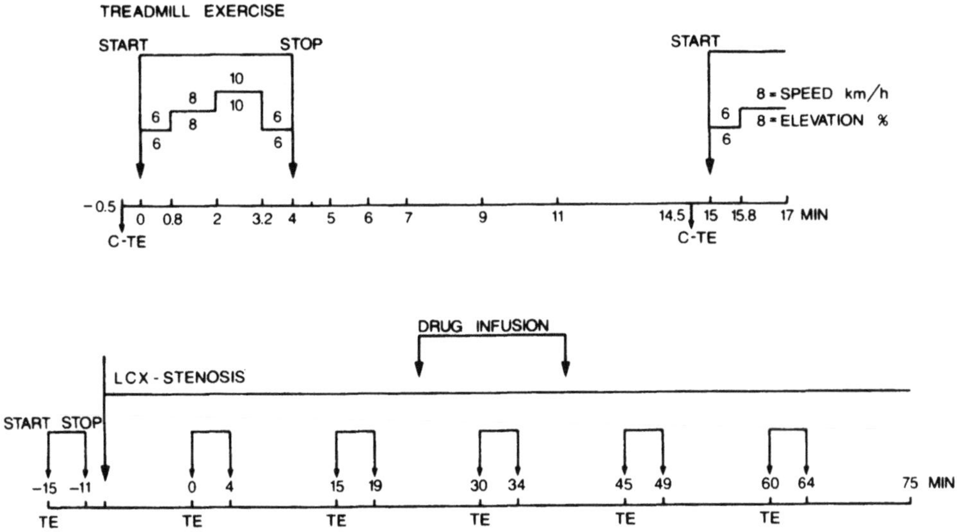

Fig. 4 Diagrammatic presentation of the treadmill exercise cycles with LCX stenosis and nitroglycerin infusion. Upper panel: treadmill exercise with different stages of speed and elevation followed by a recovery period. Lower panel: chronological arrangement of warm-up exercise, LCX stenosis and nitroglycerin infusion.

Discussion

An intravenous infusion of nitroglycerin (Nitro Pohl® infus) showed no significant effects on hemodynamics and myocardial function at rest at a dosage of 15 μg/kg/ 15 min. Only a slight decrease in systolic and diastolic arterial pressure was seen, which led to a slight increase in heart rate at rest via sympathetic counterregulation [4]. Although nitroglycerin did not provoke any significant alterations at rest, the exercise induced increase in heart rate was distinctly diminished. Since nitroglycerin has no negative chronotropic activity itself [5], the decrease in heart rate at maximum workload ($p < 0.05$) as well as the reduction in exercise induced increase in heart rate ($p < 0.01$) must be due to decreased sympathetic activity. Although sympathetic activity was reduced, left ventricular dp/dt showed an increase at maximum workload after nitroglycerin. Since myocardial dysfunction did not occur after nitroglycerin even at maximum workload ($p < 0.001$), the completely recovered function in the LCX area must be responsible for the apparent positive inotropic effect. An

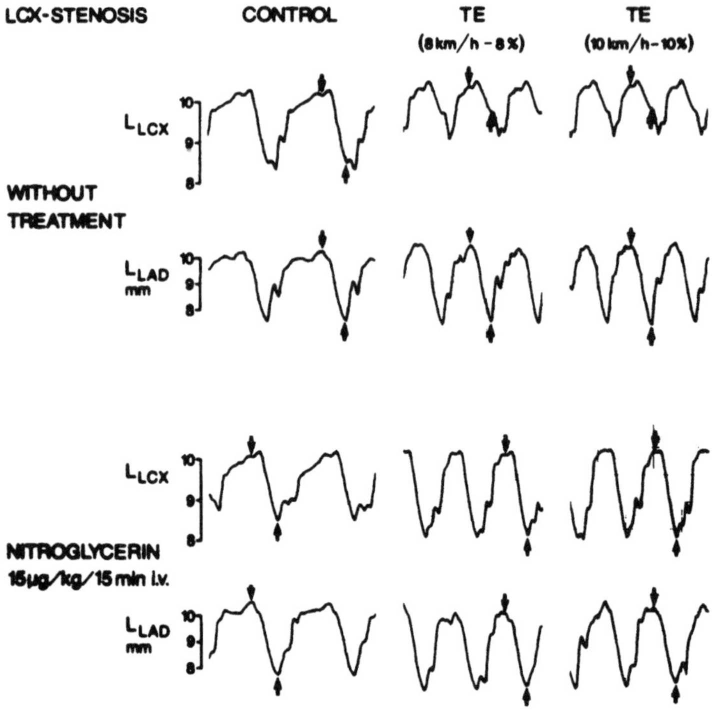

Fig. 5 Original recordings of regional myocardial shortening in the LCX- (L-LCX) and LAD area (L-LAD). Upper panel: treadmill exercise before nitroglycerin. Lower panel: treadmill exercise after nitroglycerin. ↓ : beginning of systolic shortening (= enddiastolic length); ↑ : end of systolic shortening (= endsystolic length).

In the underperfused LCX area an increase in workload leads to regional myocardial dysfunction (decrease in systolic shortening L-LCX). This contractile dysfunction in the LCX area is completely prevented by nitroglycerin (no exercise induced reduction in systolic shortening SST-LCX).

important parameter for the recovery in function is a normalized exercise induced increase in left ventricular filling pressure after nitroglycerin ($p < 0.001$), which influences the epi/endo ratio in coronary perfusion [6] by a decrease in coronary resistance. Furthermore, a reduction in ventricular dimensions [7, 8] leads to a decrease in left ventricular wall tension and thereby to a reduction in myocardial energy demand [9]. Since venous capacitance vessels show a higher sensivity for nitroglycerin than arterial resistance vessels in a therapeutic dosage range [10, 11], this improvement seems to be mainly due to venodilation (e.g. in the splanchnic

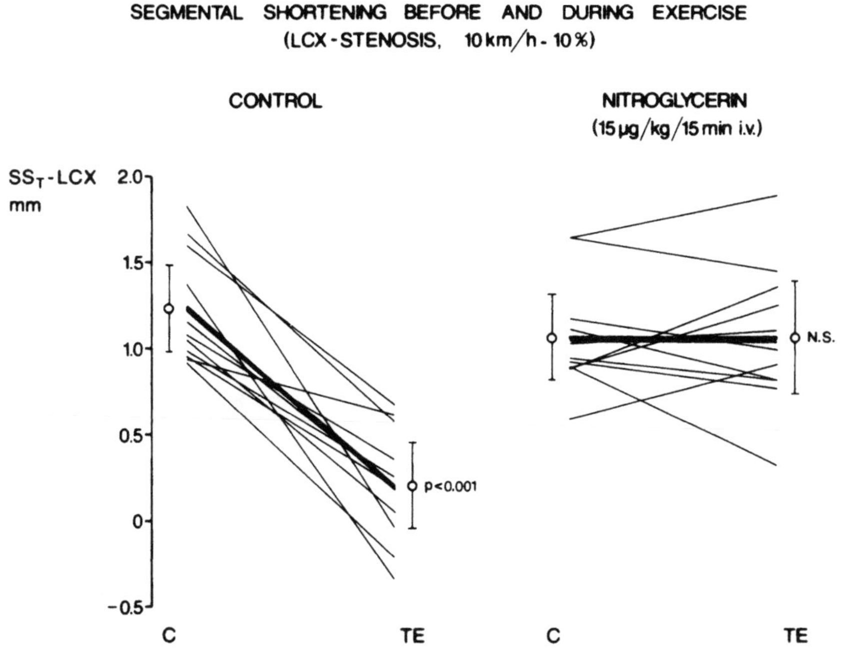

Fig. 6 Treadmill exercise with LCX stenosis, before and after nitroglycerin infusion: mean ± SD (n = 12).

Left panel: A decrease in regional systolic shortening (SST-LCX) with treadmill exercise is indicative of regional myocardial dysfunction in the underperfused LCX area. Right panel: Unaltered systolic shortening with treadmill exercise after nitroglycerin.

area) [12]. Myocardial function is restored by venous pooling [13], as well as – to a smaller extent – by facilitated ejection work against the reduced peripheral resistance. In our investigation with fixed coronary stenosis we could not elucidate to what extent an improvement in coronary collateral circulation causes an improvement in contractility after nitroglycerin [14, 15]. However, we demonstrated the cardioprotective effect of nitroglycerin used in a dosage range that does not affect hemodynamics and parameters of myocardial function at rest, but is able to prevent exercise induced myocardial dysfunction.

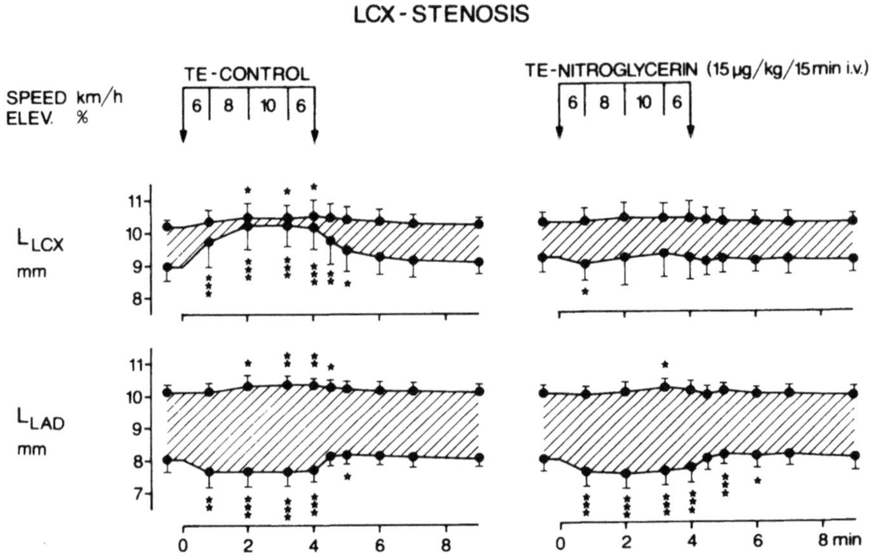

Fig. 7 Treadmill exercise with LCX stenosis, before and after nitroglycerin infusion: mean ± SD (n = 12). Segmental functional parameters at rest and during exercise.

L-LCX: segment length in the LCX area; upper curve = enddiastolic length; lower curve = endsystolic length; the height of the hatched area is equivalent to systolic shortening of the segment (SST-LCX). L-LAD = segment length in the LAD area analogous to L-LCX.

Left: The control exercise before nitroglycerin infusion shows a decrease in systolic shortening (L-LCX) in the underperfused area with treadmill exercise. Right: Prevention of regional contractile dysfunction in the LCX area after nitroglycerin.

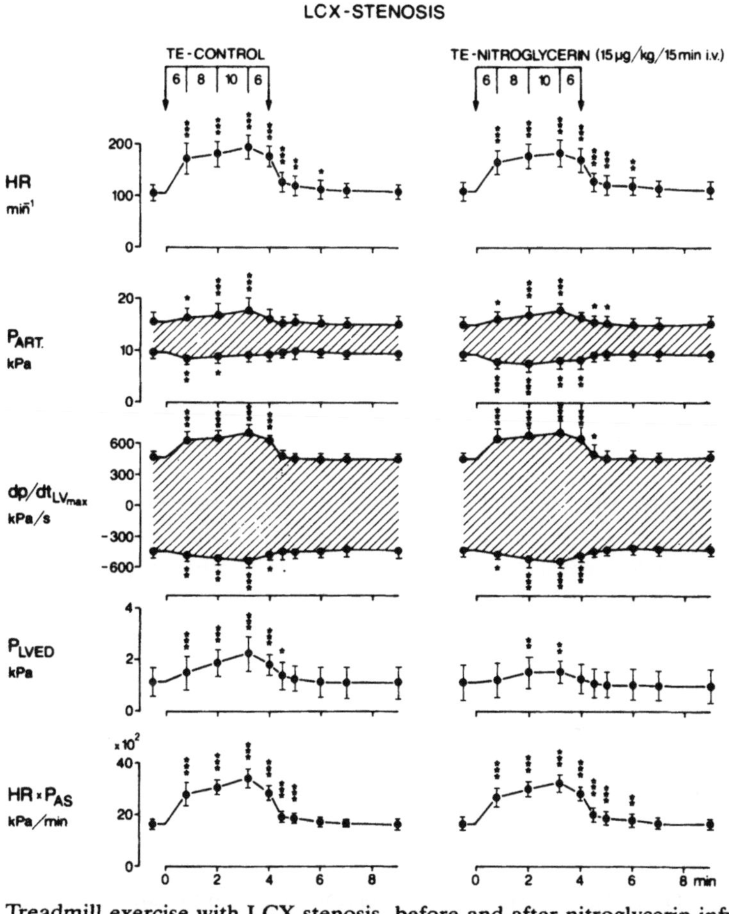

Fig. 8 Treadmill exercise with LCX stenosis, before and after nitroglycerin infusion: mean ± SD (n = 12). Hemodynamic parameters at rest and during exercise.

Left: The control exercise before nitroglycerin shows a pathological increase in P-LVED with maximal workload. Right: the exercise induced increase in P-LVED is normalized after nitroglycerin.

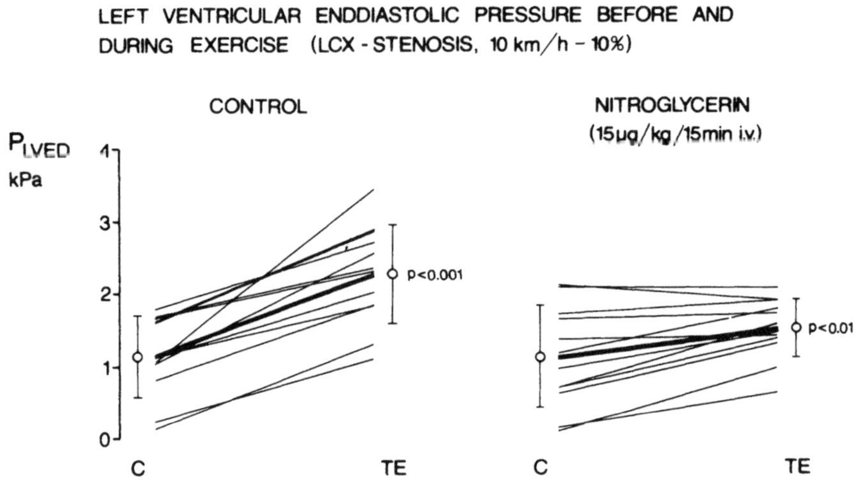

Fig. 9 Treadmill exercise with LCX stenosis, before and after nitroglycerin infusion: mean ± SD (n = 12).

Left: Increase in left ventricular enddiastolic pressure (P-LVED) to pathological values with treadmill exercise. Right: Normalized exercise induced increase after nitroglycerin.

References

[1] Seitelberger, R., G. Raberger: J. Pharmacol. Meth. **12** (1984) 233.
[2] Raberger, G., G. Krumpl, N. Mayer: J. Pharmacol. Meth. (in press).
[3] Kumada, T. et al.: Am. J. Physiol. **239** (1980) H 399.
[4] Vatner, S. F., et al.: Am. J. Physiol. (3) **234** (1978) H 244.
[5] Himori, N. et al.: Clin. Exp. Pharmacol. Physiol. **4** (1977) 257.
[6] Weiss, H. R., M. M. Winbury: Microvasc. Res. **4** (1972) 273.
[7] O'Rourke, R. A. et al.: J. Pharmacol. Exp. Ther. **177** (1971) 426.
[8] De Maria, A. N. et al.: Am. J. Med. **57** (1974) 754.
[9] Baller, D. et al.: Basic Res. Cardiol. **79** (1984) 176.
[10] Miller, R. R. et al.: Circ. Res. **39** (1976) 127.
[11] Mackenzie, J. E., J. R. Parrat: Br. J. Pharmacol. **60** (1977) 155.
[12] Smith, E. R. et al.: Am. J. Med. **76** (1984) 14.
[13] Strauer, B. E., A. Scherpe: Am. Heart J. **95** (1978) 210.
[14] Weintraub, W. S. et al.: Cardiovasc. Res. **19** (1985) 169.
[15] Sakamoto, S., M. Yokoyama, H. Fukuzaki: J. Cardiovasc. Pharmacol. **7** (1985) 562.

Prevention of diminished activity of glyceryl trinitrate by use of an aerosol

K. K. Teo, J. H. Horgan

Sublingual glyceryl trinitrate remains a major therapy for the rapid relief of angina pectoris.

However, a recent study has shown that significant loss of activity occurs as a result of poor patient compliance with storage instructions [1]. We, therefore, evaluated the stability of an aerosol preparation that has been shown to be therapeutically effective [2].

Glyceryl trinitrate aerosol, manufactured in April, 1979 (A) and March, 1982 (B), was administered to 10 volunteers, mean age 25.8 ± 2.9 years (± standard deviation). The glyceryl trinitrate was stored dissolved in an absorbable oily base in sealed pressured canisters and 0.4 mg was administered on to the buccal mucosa or sublingually. Each volunteer randomly received A, B or placebo on a double blind fashion on 3 consecutive days.

Heart rates were determined from electrocardiographic tracings and blood pressures were automatically measured by an infrasonde electric blood pressure monitor (model D 400) in order to overcome intraobserver error. Three measurements were made at 2-minute intervals to establish a steady baseline before treatment. Repeat observations were made immediately after and at 2-minute intervals for 10 minutes, then at 5-minute intervals for the succeeding 20 minutes and 10-minute intervals for the final 30 minutes (fig. 1).

Changes in heart rates and blood pressures were compared using paired T tests and areas under the heart rate-time curves were calculated by the trapezoidal rule.

The area under the heart rate-time curves for both, estimated from the time of drug administration for up to 15, 20, 30 and 40 minutes, did not show significant differences. Blood pressures did not change significantly with either active agent or placebo. Three objects noted mild headache with aerosol A and 4 with aerosol B, all within 10 minutes after administration.

The average changes in heart rates produced by each of the agents are as shown in figure 1. Both aerosol A and B produced increases in heart rates, whereas this was not so with placebo. The differences between the changes in heart rates for both,

Nitroglycerin 5

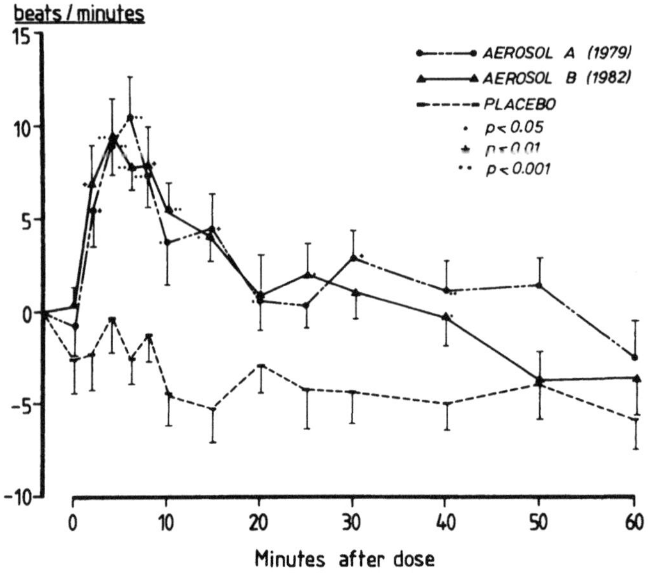

Fig. 1 Change in heart rate.

compared with placebo, were consistently significant from 2 minutes and up to 20 minutes for A ($p \leq 0.01$) and 15 minutes for B ($p \leq 0.01$). Significant differences could still be demonstrated for up to 40 minutes.

Glyceryl trinitrate, presented as an aerosol, has been shown to be effective and thus presented it may obviate the problems of improper storage and instability which attend the use of glyceryl trinitrate tablets.

References

[1] O'Hanrahan, M., K. Mc Garry, J. G. Kelly et al.: Diminished activity of glyceryl trinitrate. Br. Med. J. **284** (1982) 1183–1186.

[2] Kimchi, A., G. Lee, E. Amsterdam et al.: Increased exercise tolerance after nitroglycerin oral spray: a new and effective therapeutic modality in angina pectoris. Circulation **67** (1983) 124–127.

Contrasting effects of Nitrolingual-Spray® at rest and after exercise induced angina post exercise on myocardial nutrient flow

I. Hutton, A. C. Tweddel, I. McGhie, W. Martin

Introduction

In 1867 Lauder Brunton [1] first used amyl nitrate to "lessen the arterial tension" in a patient with nocturnal angina. He had observed that venesection was an effective method of pain relief and it was in an effort to spare his patients repeated "bleedings" that he introduced nitrate. More recently Brown [2] has demonstrated a direct dilation effect of nitrate on the occlusive lesion in coronary arteries. Nitrates also have an effect on ventricular function, reducing end diastolic and end systolic wall tension [3]. This effect is augmented by reduced venous return, leading to a fall in end-diastolic volume and thus overall tension, and reduced myocardial oxygen consumption. In addition an arteriolar dilatory effect leads to a reduction in afterload. The peripheral action of nitrate was emphasised by Ganz and Marcus [4] who found that pacing induced angina was relieved by intravenous and not by intracoronary nitroglycerin administration.

The purpose of this study was to determine the effect of sublingual nitrate on regional myocardial nutrient flow at rest and following symptom limited dynamic exercise in patients with coronary heart disease.

Methods

A total of 51 patients were studied – 35 at rest and 16 immediately post dynamic exercise. 10 patients had normal coronary arteries and 41 significant obstructive coronary disease, defined as a 50% or greater reduction in luminal diameter of any major epicardial vessel. The mean age of the group was 52 years with an age range of 37–65 years. 42 patients were male and 9 female. All cardioactive drug therapy was withdrawn 24 hours prior to the study, and long-acting nitrate preparations were withdrawn for a period of 48 hours. Informed consent was obtained from all patients and approval was obtained from the Ethical Committee of the Glasgow Royal Infirmary. The detailed clinical information is found in table 1.

Nitroglycerin 5

Table 1

Total 51 patients	– 41 significant coronary artery disease	
	– 10 normal vessels	
Studied at rest	– 35 patients – 26 male, 9 female	
10 normal vessels		21 LAD
6 single vessel involvement		18 RCA
11 double vessel involvement		13 Cx
8 triple vessel involvement		Total 52 diseased vessels
Studied post exercise	– 16 patients, males	
4 single vessel involvement		14 LAD
5 double vessel involvement		13 RCA
7 triple vessel involvement		8 Cx
	Total	35 diseased vessels

LAD = left anterior descending artery
RCA = right coronary artery
Cx = Circumflex coronary artery

Cardiac catheterisation

Patients were predmedicated with 10 mg of oral diazepam. The femoral artery was cannulated percutaneously, leaving a sheath in situ for ease of changing catheters. Biplane left ventriculography was performed during held inspiration using 40 mls of iopamidol injected over 2.5 seconds. A 2 centimeter square grid was filmed for each patient as spatial reference for magnification correction. Regional wall motion was assessed visually and ejection fraction was calculated in the 30° right anterior oblique projection by the method of Sandler and Dodge [5]. Selective coronary arteriograms were obtained in multiple views pre and post intracoronary nitrate and analysed independently by 2 observers. Reductions in luminal diameter of coronary arteries and the presence of collaterals were assessed and graded visually.

Myocardial nutrient flow

Myocardial nutrient flow was measured using a Xenon clearance technique. At least 30 minutes following ventriculography and coronary arteriography, $Xenon_{133}$ was injected intracoronary under direct vision into each coronary ostium, with the image intensifier in the right anterior oblique projection. A bolus of Xenon, made up to 0.5 ml with saline, was preloaded into the catheter and flushed with 1.5 to 2.0 ml of saline. Xenon injections which induced electrocardiographic change were rejected. Incremental doses of Xenon to a total of 800 MBq were employed to obviate the problems of background and at least 10 minutes were allowed to elapse between resting injection and those post exercise, thus allowing lung clearance. Myocardial activity was imaged using a mobile Gamma camera (General Electrics) in the 30–40° left anterior oblique projection, with an ultra high sensitivity parallel collimeter. The data were processed using a mobile computer (Link Systems MAPS), and analysis of the washout curves was made by applying a mono-exponential model to the initial 30 seconds of data according to the Kety formula [6].

$$F = \frac{100 \times K \times \lambda}{P} \text{ mls/min/100 g}$$

Where F is the myocardial nutrient flow in millilitres per 100 grams of myocardium per minute.

λ = the myocardium: blood partition coefficient obtained by Conn [7] in normal dog (.072).

P = the specific gravity of the heart (1.05)

and

K = the rate constant derived from a least squares fit of the monoexponential to the first 30 seconds of data.

Mean left ventricular flows, corrected for distribution were calculated for each patient, and are termed weighted flows.

Regions of interest were drawn, 8 for the left ventricular myocardium and 3 over the right ventricle. Normal distribution and regional nutrient flow had been previously determined for both right and left dominant systems in patients with arteriographically normal coronary arteries and atypical chest pain, and from the patients with normal vessels included in this study. The reproducibility of these measurements was ±8%. From the left coronary injections, three regions were allocated to the left anterior descending territory and three posterior regions to the circumflex distribution. From the right coronary injection the three right ventricular regions and two inferior left ventricular regions were designated to the right coronary artery. Regions of distribution and flow identified outwith the normal for either right or left dominant circulation were termed "collateral flow" i.e. distribution to the inferior surface from the left coronary injection or to either the septum and/or posteriorly from the right coronary injection. Mean flow from each of the left ventricular territories are presented, rather than individual regions.

In 35 patients, control data was obtained from both the right and left coronary arteries. A metered dose of 0.4 mg nitrolingual nitrate spray was administered, and the right coronary injection repeated at 120 seconds. After 10–15 minutes, or longer if haemodynamic measurements had not returned to control, the catheter was changed and a further 0.4 mg spray of sublingual nitrate was followed by a further left coronary injection at 120 seconds.

In 16 patients, resting control data were obtained from both arteries. Patients performed maximal symptom limited exercise on a supine bicycle ergometer, fixed to the catherisation table. Repeat coronary injection was performed immediately post exercise, first to the left coronary artery, then the right coronary artery. The patient was rested supine for 1 hour, and the above procedure was repeated, but on this occasion a metered dose of 0.4 mg nitrolingual nitrate spray was administered immediately on stopping exercise, when the patient developed angina.

Exercise tests

Maximal symptom limited exercise tests were performed on an upright bicycle ergometer, the day prior to the study. A continuous multistage protocol was employed, with 50 watt increments in workload. The electrocardiogram was monitored continuously with a modified v_5 electrode position, and intermittent sampling of electrocardiogram and cuff blood pressure. Horizontal or down-sloping ST depression of 0.1 millivolt with a duration of 80 milliseconds past the j-point was considered a positive test. At the time of cardiac catheterisation, maximal symptom limited exercise tests were performed with the same multistage protocol, using a supine bicycle ergometer. A 6 lead standard electrocardiogram was monitored continuously and intra-aortic pressure was obtained from the femoral catheter.

Statistical analysis

Results are expressed as means with standard error of the mean shown. Statistical significance was obtained by applying the Wilcoxon paired and group test as appropriate.

Results

Patients studied at rest

35 patients were studied, of whom 10 had arteriographically normal vessels, 6 single, 11 double and 8 triple vessel involvement. None had left main stem disease. This gave a total of 52 diseased vessels, of which 21 were left anterior descending, 18 right coronary artery and 13 circumflex coronary artery.

At rest 0.4 mg nitrolingual nitrate produced a mean increase in heart rate of 2 beats/min, and mean arterial pressure fell by 7 mmHg (87 ± 3 to 80 ± 3 mmHg).

Sublingual nitrate increased flow in arteriographically normal arteries; left anterior descending increasing from 42 ± 10 to 45 ± 9 ml/100 gm/min, right coronary artery left centricular flow increasing from 30 ± 4.5 to 37 ± 7 ml/100 gm/min ($p < 0.01$) and circumflex from 57 ± 9 to 62 ± 14 ml/100 gm/min (fig. 1).

In regions subtended by arteries with high grade occlusions myocardial nutrient flow fell, following nitrate administration. In regions supplied by the left anterior descending by 19% ($p < 0.01$), right coronary artery 17% ($p < 0.01$) and circumflex by 7%. In those regions supplied by 'collaterals' nutrient flow fell by 27% ($p < 0.05$) (figs. 2 and 3).

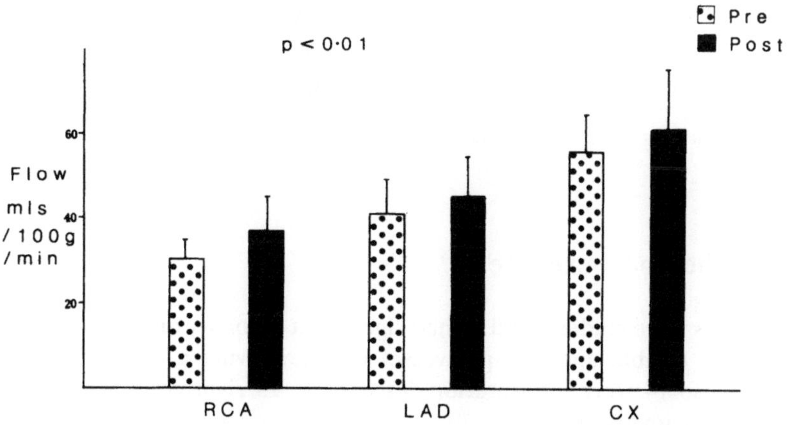

Fig. 1 Effect of sublingual nitrate on arteriographically normal vessels. RCA = right coronary artery. LAD = left anterior descending coronary artery. Cx = circumflex coronary artery.

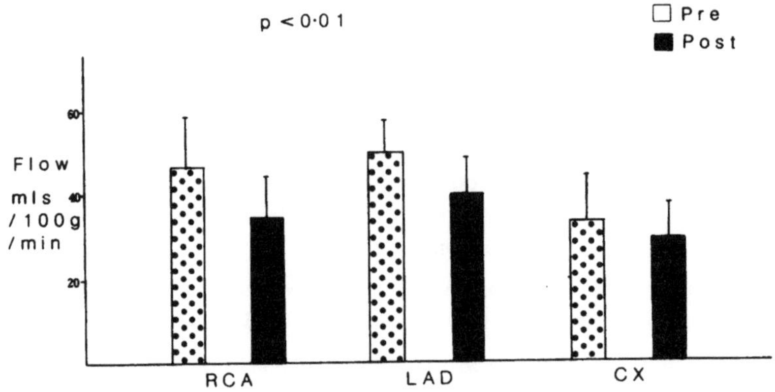

Fig. 2 Effect of sublingual nitrate on abnormal coronary vessels. RCA = right coronary artery. LAD = left anterior descending coronary artery. Cx = circumflex coronary artery.

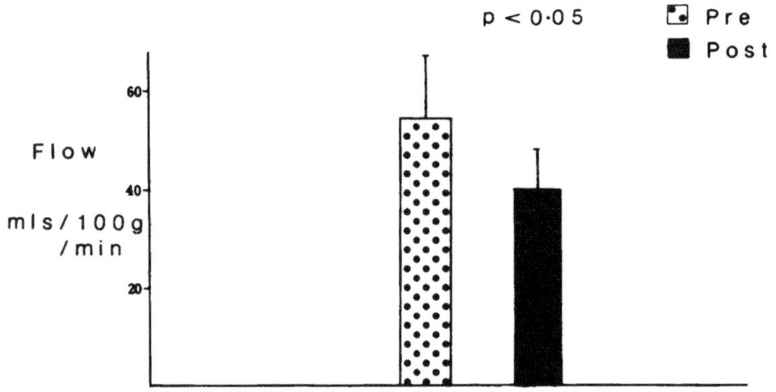

Fig. 3 Effect of sublingual nitrate on "collateral" distributions.

Patients studied post-exercise

16 male patients were studied, and all had significant coronary disease, 4 single vessel involvement, 5 double and 7 triple vessel disease, giving a total of 35 diseased vessels. Of these 14 were left anterior descending, 13 right coronary artery and 8 circumflex artery involvement.

Heart rate and intra-arterial pressure were measured at rest and during exercise. Control and peak exercise values are seen in table 2, and were similar on both occasions. Symptomatic end points did not change; in 15 patients this was angina on both occasions and in 1 dyspnoea with marked ST depression on the electrocardiogram. Time to angina (256 ± 24.6 and 264 ± 23.4 seconds) and maximal work load (96.8 ± 8.5 and 100 ± 8.0 watts) were similar.

Immediately post exercise, mean left ventricular nutrient flow was increased in areas supplied by diseased arteries, although mean percentage increase of 20% was less than in patients with normal vessels (> 50%). Mean left ventricular weighted flow increased from 48.2 ± 12.9% to 89.4 ± 19.0 ml/100 gm/min ($p < 0.001$) (tab. 3).

Table 2 Exercise haemodynamics

	Control	Nitrate
Resting heart rate (beats/min)	63.5 ± 2.1	65.1 ± 2.6
Resting mean arterial pressure (mmHg)	96.3 ± 2.4	96.4 ± 2.3
Exercise heart rate (beats/min)	89.4 ± 4.5	85.8 ± 3.3
Exercise mean arterial pressure (mmHg)	116.8 ± 4.1	119.3 ± 3.4
Work Load (watts)	96.8 ± 8.5	100.0 ± 8.0
Time to symptoms (S)	256.0 ± 24.6	264.0 ± 23.4

Table 3 Exercise nutrient flow

Nutrient flow (ml/100mg/min) increasing on exercise					
Distribution	*n*	*Mean flow at rest*	*Mean flow exercise*	*Mean diff.*	*P.*
LAD	13	37.3 ± 3.9	57.9 ± 6.0	20.6 ± 5.1	< 0.001
RCA	5	22.4 ± 6.7	30.6 ± 5.7	8.2 ± 3.3	
Cx	8	38.6 ± 6.9	61.5 ± 5.8	19.9 ± 3.8	< 0.05
Seen only on exercise (RCA)	5	0	9.2 ± 1.7		< 0.01
Nutrient flow (ml/100 gm/min) falling or unchanged on exercise					
Distribution	*n*	*Mean flow at rest*	*Mean flow exercise*	*Mean difference*	
LAD	1	41.0	41.0	0	
RCA	2	75.0 ± 2.0	64.0 ± 1.0	11.0 ± 1.0	
Cx	–	–	–	–	

LAD = left anterior descending coronary artery
RCA = right coronary artery
Cx = circumflex coronary artery
Diff = difference

With nitrate in the left anterior descending distribution, post exercise flow was slightly higher (mean difference rest to exercise 22.5 ± 5.4 ml/100 gm/min (vs 20.6 ± 5.1 ml/100 gm/min)), where flow increased in response to exercise. However in 2 patients, with nitrate, flow fell post exercise (mean difference – 9 ± 2 ml/100 gm/min). In the region of the right coronary artery, a similar pattern was seen. Nitrate administration increased post exercise in 3 regions (mean difference rest to exercise 19 ± 12.9 ml/100 gm/min), but in 6 regions flow fell post exercise (mean difference −7.8 ± 3.8 ml/100 gm/min). In the distribution supplied by diseased circumflex vessels, flow was little affected by nitrate (mean difference rest to exercise 19.9 ± 3.8 and 21.5 ± 2.9 ml/100 gm/min with nitrate) (tab. 4).

Overall in 26 distributions, nutrient flow increased in response to exercise (mean difference 18.0 ± 4.2 ml/100 mg/min) and with nitrate, this increased further to 21.7 ± 7.1 ml/100 mg/min. In addition, five regions of supply were seen only post exercise. Post control exercise, flow fell in only 3 regions (mean difference −11 ± 1 ml/100 gm/min) but with nitrate administration, flow fell in 7 regions (mean difference −8.4 ± 2.9 ml/100 mg/min).

Table 4 Effect of nitrolingual on exercise flow

Nutrient flow (ml/100 gm/min) increasing on exercise					
Distribution	*n*	*Mean flow at rest*	*Mean flow on exercise*	*Mean diff.*	*P.*
LAD	12	32.8 ± 3.5	55.3 ± 5.9	22.5 ± 5.4	< 0.001
RCA	3	23.0 ± 4.8	42.0 ± 9.0	19.0 ± 12.9	
Cx	8	43.1 ± 5.2	64.6 ± 6.3	21.5 ± 2.9	< 0.01
Seen only on exercise	1	0	6		
Nutrient flow (ml/100 gm/min) falling or unchanged on exercise					
Distribution	*n*	*Mean flow at rest*	*Mean flow on exercise*	*Mean difference*	
LAD	2	62.0 ± 12.0	53.0 ± 9.0	9.0 ± 2.0	
RCA	6	24.0 ± 7.0	16.2 ± 3.81	7.8 ± 3.8	
Cx	0	–	–	–	
No flow at rest or on exercise (RCA)					

LAD = left anterior descending coronary artery
RCA = right coronary artery
Cx = circumflex coronary artery
Diff = difference

"Collateral flow"

A total of 22 "collateral" distributions were identified by Xenon of which 11 were seen angiographically; 8 to left anterior descending, 10 to right coronary artery and 4 to circumflex distributions. With exercise mean flow increased from 38.8 ± 6.3 to 50.5 ± 10.5 ml/100 gm/min. With the second post exercise scan, following nitrate, mean flow increased from 35.8 ± 5.7 to 43.3 ± 5.9 ml/100 gm/min and one further collateral distribution was identified post nitrate, which had not been seen either at rest or with the control exercise scan.

In 8 "collateral" distributions, nutrient flow fell in response to exercise (mean difference rest to exercise 15.6 ± 7.8 ml/100 gm/min) and with nitrate this was further reduced to a mean of 12.4 ± 3.4 ml/100 gm/min. Myocardial flow increased post exercise in 14 "collateral" distributions (mean difference 27/2 ± 11.6 ml/100 gm/min) and with nitrate mean difference fell to 23.0 ± 4.8 ml/100 gm/min (tab. 5).

Discussion

This study shows that at rest sublingual nitrate appears to compromise regions of myocardial flow, supplied by vessels with high grade occlusions, or by collateral flow. As no patient developed chest pain or electrocardiographic evidence of myocardial ischaemia this would suggest that myocardial oxygen demand was reduced, presumably by a peripheral action on venous capacitance vessels.

The net effect of nitrate given immediately after the onset of angina was to increase nutrient flow, both in regions subtended by diseased vessels and where the myocardium was supplied by collaterals. From previous work [8], the ability of a region to increase flow in response to exercise is not necessarily related either to the degree of

Table 5 "Collateral flow" (ml/100 gm/ min)

	n	*Mean flow at rest*		*Mean flow on exercise*
Control	22	38.8 ± 6.3		50.5 ± 10.5
With nitrate	22	35.8 ± 5.7		43.3 ± 5.9
Response to exercise; mean difference in flow ml/100 gm/min				
	n	*Control*	*n*	*With nitrate*
Increasing with exercise	14	27.2 ± 11.6	13	23.0 ± 4.8
Decreasing with exercise	8	15.6 ± 7.8	9	12.4 ± 3.4

disease in the subtending vessel, or where collaterals are involved, where the area is supplied by a "compromised" or "non-compromised" collateral [9]. Similar mixed results were reported by Horowitz et al. [10] who stressed the myocardium using isoproterenol infusions. Presumably the response to stress in any one region is related both to the myocardial oxygen demand and the vasodilatory reserve of that region [11]. Previously we have shown [8] that the ability of collateral flow to increase in response to exercise is associated with preserved regional left ventricular function.

In this study a relatively small dose of nitrate was used 0.4 mg but it is the dose which is used normally by patients. Haemodynamic changes were small and this possible explains some of the difference in findings between our study in patients at rest and those of others [15, 16].

In conclusion this study has demonstrated that the changes in myocardial nutrient flow following the administration of nitrate to patients with coronary heart disease who are asymptomatic, bears little relation to the effects of nitrate given to relieve exercise induced angina. Nitrate in many patients can increase myocardial nutrient flow when given sublingually to relieve the symptoms of exercise induced angina.

References

[1] Brunton, T. L.: On the use of nitrate of amyl in angina pectoris. Lancet **2** (1867) 97.

[2] Brown, B. G.: Vasodilatation of coronarx stenosis as one of the major components of the beneficial effects of glyceryl trinitrate. Br. J. Clinic. Pract., Suppl. **26** (1982) 45–52.

[3] Greenberg, H., E. M. Dwyer, A. G. Jameson et al.: Effects of nitroglycerin on the major determinants of myocardial oxygen consumption. Am. J. Cardiol. **36** (1975) 426–432.

[4] Ganz, W., H. S. Marcus: Failure of intracoronary nitroglycerin to alleviate pacing-induced angina. Circulation **XLVI** (1972) 880–889.

[5] Sandler, H., H. T. Dodge: The use of single plane angiocardiogram for the calculation of left ventricular volume in man. Am. Heart J. **75** (1968) 325.

[6] Kety, S.: The theory and applications of the exchange of inert gas at the lungs and tissue. Pharmacol. Rev. **3** (1951) 1–41.

[7] Conn, H. L.: Equilibrium distribution of radioxenon in tissue-xenon-haemoglobin association curve. J. Appl. Physiol. **16** (1960) 1065–1070.

[8] Tweddel, A. C., W. Martin, I. McGhie et al.: Impact on left ventricular function of the exercise response of coronary collateral flow in coronary heart disease. J. Nucl. Med. 1985 (in press).

[9] Eng, C., R. E. Patterson, S. F. Horowitz et al.: Coronary collateral function during exercise. Circulation **2** (1982) 309–315.

[10] Horowitz, L. D., G. C. Curry, R. W. Parkey et al.: Differentiation of physiologically significant coronary artery lesions by coronary blood flow measurements during isoproterenol infusion. Circulation **XLIX** (1974) 55–62.

[11] Klocke, F. J.: Measurements of coronary blood flow and degree of stenosis: Current clinical implications and continuing uncertainties. J. Am. Coll Cardiol. **1** (1983) 31–41.
[12] Matsuda, Y., H. Ogawa, K. Moritani et al.: Transient appearances of collateral during vasospastic occlusion in patients without obstructive coronary atherosclerosis. Am. Heart. J. **4** (1985) 759–763.
[13] Retrop, P., M. Cohen, H. Blanke et al.: Changes in collateral channel filling immediately after controlled coronary artery occlusion by an angioplasty balloon in human subjects. JACC **3** (1985) 587–592.
[14] Brown, B. G., E. Polson, R. B. Petersen et al.: The mechanisms of nitroglycerin action: stenosis vasodilatation as a major component of the drug response. Circulation **6** (1981) 1089–1100.
[15] Parker, J. O., R. O. West, S. Di Giorgi: The effect of nitroglycerin on coronary blood flow and the haemodynamic response to exercise in coronary artery disease. Am. J. Cardiol. **17** (1971) 59–65.
[16] Cohn, P. F., O. Maddox, B. L. Holnan et al.: Effect of sublingually administered nitroglycerin on regional myocardial blood low in patients with coronary artery disease. Am. J. Cardiol. **39** (1977) 672–678.
[17] Cannon, P. J., R. R. Sciacca, D. L. Fowler et al.: Measurement of regional myocardial blood flow in man. Description on critique of the method using Xenon-133 and a scintillation camera. Am. J. Cardiol. **36** (1975) 783–792.